Psychopharmacology and Psychobiology of Ethnicity

PROGRESS IN PSYCHIATRY

Number 39
David Spiegel, M.D.
Series Editor

Psychopharmacology and Psychobiology of Ethnicity

Edited by
Keh-Ming Lin, M.D., M.P.H.
Russell E. Poland, Ph.D.
Gayle Nakasaki, M.S.W.

American Psychiatric Press, Inc.

Washington, DC
London, England

Note: The authors have worked to ensure that all information in this book concerning drug dosages, schedules, and routes of administration is accurate as of the time of publication and consistent with standards set by the U.S. Food and Drug Administration and the general medical community. As medical research and practice advance, however, therapeutic standards may change. For this reason and because human and mechanical errors sometimes occur, we recommend that readers follow the advice of a physician who is directly involved in their care or the care of a member of their family.

Manufactured in the United States of America on acid-free paper
First Edition 96 95 94 93 4 3 2 1
American Psychiatric Press, Inc.
1400 K Street, N.W., Washington, DC 20005

Library of Congress Cataloging-in-Publication Data
Psychopharmacology and psychobiology of ethnicity / edited by
Keh-Ming Lin, Russell E. Poland, Gayle Nakasaki.
p. cm. — (Progress in psychiatry series : [#39])
Includes bibliographical references and index.
ISBN 0-88048-471-3
1. Psychopharmacology—Cross-cultural studies. 2. Mental illness—Genetic aspects—Cross-cultural studies. 3. Biochemical markers—Cross-cultural studies. I. Lin, Keh-Ming, 1946– . II. Poland, Russell E., 1946– . III. Nakasaki, Gayle, 1963– . IV. Series.
[DNLM: 1. Biological Markers. 2. Ethnic Groups. 3. Mental Disorders—drug therapy. 4. Mental Disorders—ethnology. 5. Psychotropic Drugs—therapeutic use. W1 PR6781L no.39 / / WM 100 P989445]
RC455.4.B5P795 1993
615'.78'089—dc20
DNLM/DLC
for Library of Congress 92-49996
CIP

British Library Cataloguing in Publication Data
A CIP record is available from the British Library.

Contents

Section II
Ethnicity and Psychopharmacology

Section III
Ethnicity and Psychobiology

Contributors

Linda Chang, M.S., M.D.
Assistant Professor of Neurology, UCLA, Department of Neurology, Harbor-UCLA Medical Center, Torrance, California

Wen-Ho Chang, M.D.
Chief, Laboratory of Biological Psychiatry, Taipei City Psychiatric Center, Taipei, Taiwan

Joseph C. Fleishaker, Ph.D.
Senior Research Scientist, Clinical Pharmacokinetics Unit, Pharmaceutical Research and Development, The Upjohn Company, Kalamazoo, Michigan

Paul Fu, Ph.D.
Professor of Pathology, UCLA, Department of Pathology, Harbor-UCLA Medical Center, Torrance, California

Gregory E. Gray, M.D., Ph.D.
Associate Professor of Clinical Psychiatry and Preventive Medicine, University of Southern California; Director, Adult Psychiatric Inpatient Service, Los Angeles County/University of Southern California Medical Center, Los Angeles, California

Mary A. Gutierrez, Pharm.D.
Assistant Professor of Clinical Pharmacy, University of Southern California School of Pharmacy, Los Angeles, California

Tadanobu Inaba, Ph.D.
Professor of Pharmacology, Department of Pharmacology, Faculty of Medicine, University of Toronto, Toronto, Ontario, Canada

Michael W. Jann, Pharm.D.
Associate Professor, Mercer University, Southern School of Pharmacy, Atlanta, Georgia

Werner Kalow, M.D., F.R.S.C.
Professor Emeritus, Department of Pharmacology, University of Toronto, Toronto, Ontario, Canada

Y. W. Francis Lam, Pharm.D.
Assistant Professor, College of Pharmacy, The University of Texas at Austin, Austin, Texas, and the University of Texas Health Science Center at San Antonio, San Antonio, Texas

William Lawson, M.D., Ph.D.
Associate Professor of Psychiatry, Department of Psychiatry, University of Arkansas School of Medicine, Little Rock, Arkansas; Chief Assistant, Veteran Administration Medical Center in Arkansas, North Little Rock, Arkansas

Keh-Ming Lin, M.D., M.P.H.
Associate Professor of Psychiatry, UCLA, Department of Psychiatry and Research Center on the Psychobiology of Ethnicity, Harbor-UCLA Medical Center, Research and Education Institute, Inc., Torrance, California

Ricardo Mendoza, M.D.
Associate Clinical Professor of Psychiatry, UCLA, Department of Psychiatry and Research Center on the Psychobiology of Ethnicity, Harbor-UCLA Medical Center, Research and Education Institute, Inc., Torrance, California

Bruce L. Miller, M.D.
Associate Professor of Neurology, UCLA, Department of Neurology, Harbor-UCLA Medical Center, Torrance, California

Hector F. Myers, Ph.D.
Professor, Department of Psychology, University of California, Los Angeles; Director, Biobehavioral Laboratory, Department of Psychiatry, Charles R. Drew University of Medicine and Science, Los Angeles, California

Gayle Nakasaki, M.S.W.
Assistant Director, Research Center on the Psychobiology of Ethnicity, Harbor-UCLA Medical Center, Research and Education Institute, Inc., Torrance, California

J. Paul Phillips
Senior Medical Associate, Clinical Pharmacokinetics Unit, Pharmaceutical Research and Development, The Upjohn Company, Kalamazoo, Michigan

Edmond H. Pi, M.D.
Director, Transcultural Psychiatry and Professor of Clinical Psychiatry, University of Southern California School of Medicine, Los Angeles, California

Russell E. Poland, Ph.D.
Research Pharmacologist, UCLA, Department of Psychiatry and Research Center on the Psychobiology of Ethnicity, Harbor-UCLA Medical Center, Research and Education Institute, Inc., Torrance, California

Morikazu Shibasaki, M.D.
Lecturer, Department of Psychiatry, Shiga University of Medical Science, Seta-Tsukinowa, Otsu-shi, Shiga-ken, Japan

Barbara Silver, M.D.
Assistant Professor of Psychiatry, UCLA, Department of Psychiatry and Research Center on the Psychobiology of Ethnicity, Harbor-UCLA Medical Center, Research and Education Institute, Inc., Torrance, California

Michael Smith, M.D.
Third-Year Resident, Department of Psychiatry, Harbor-UCLA Medical Center, Torrance, California

Toshiyuki Someya, M.D.
Lecturer, Department of Psychiatry, Shiga University of Medical Science, Seta-Tsukinowa, Otsu-shi, Shiga-ken, Japan

Tony L. Strickland, Ph.D.
Associate Professor of Psychiatry, UCLA and Charles R. Drew University of Medicine and Science; Associate Director of Biobehavioral Laboratory, Department of Psychiatry and Human Behavior, Charles R. Drew University of Medicine and Science, Los Angeles, California

Saburo Takahashi, M.D.
Professor and Chair, Department of Psychiatry, Shiga University of Medical Science, Seta-Tsukinowa, Otsu-shi, Shiga-ken, Japan

Siu-Wa Tang, M.D.
Chief of Psychiatry, Long Beach Veteran Administration Medical Center, Long Beach, California; Professor of Psychiatry, University of California at Irvine, Irvine, California

Akira Yoshida, Ph.D.
Director, Department of Biochemical Genetics, Beckman Research Institute of the City of Hope, Duarte, California

Introduction to the Progress in Psychiatry Series

The Progress in Psychiatry Series is designed to capture in print the excitement that comes from assembling a diverse group of experts from various locations to examine in detail the newest information about a developing aspect of psychiatry. This series emerged as a collaboration between the American Psychiatric Association's (APA) Scientific Program Committee and the American Psychiatric Press, Inc. Great interest is generated by a number of the symposia presented each year at the APA annual meeting, and we realized that much of the information presented there, carefully assembled by people who are deeply immersed in a given area, would unfortunately not appear together in print. The symposia sessions at the annual meetings provide an unusual opportunity for experts who otherwise might not meet on the same platform to share their diverse viewpoints for a period of 3 hours. Some new themes are repeatedly reinforced and gain credence, while in other instances disagreements emerge, enabling the audience and now the reader to reach informed decisions about new directions in the field. The Progress in Psychiatry Series allows us to publish and capture some of the best of the symposia and thus provide an in-depth treatment of specific areas that might not otherwise be presented in broader review formats.

Psychiatry is by nature an interface discipline, combining the study of mind and brain, of individual and social environments, of the humane and the scientific. Thus, progress in the field is rarely linear—it often comes from unexpected sources. Further, new developments emerge from an array of viewpoints that do not necessarily provide immediate agreement but rather expert examination of the issues. We intend to present innovative ideas and data that will enable you, the reader, to participate in this process.

We believe the Progress in Psychiatry Series will provide you with an opportunity to review timely new information in specific fields of interest as they are developing. We hope you find that the excitement of the presentations is captured in the written word and that this book proves to be informative and enjoyable reading.

David Spiegel, M.D.
Series Editor
Progress in Psychiatry Series

Progress in Psychiatry Series Titles

The Borderline: Current Empirical Research (#1)
Edited by Thomas H. McGlashan, M.D.

Premenstrual Syndrome: Current Findings and Future Directions (#2)
Edited by Howard J. Osofsky, M.D., Ph.D., and Susan J. Blumenthal, M.D.

Treatment of Affective Disorders in the Elderly (#3)
Edited by Charles A. Shamoian, M.D.

Post-Traumatic Stress Disorder in Children (#4)
Edited by Spencer Eth, M.D., and Robert S. Pynoos, M.D., M.P.H.

The Psychiatric Implications of Menstruation (#5)
Edited by Judith H. Gold, M.D., F.R.C.P.C.

Can Schizophrenia Be Localized in the Brain? (#6)
Edited by Nancy C. Andreasen, M.D., Ph.D.

Medical Mimics of Psychiatric Disorders (#7)
Edited by Irl Extein, M.D., and Mark S. Gold, M.D.

Biopsychosocial Aspects of Bereavement (#8)
Edited by Sidney Zisook, M.D.

Psychiatric Pharmacosciences of Children and Adolescents (#9)
Edited by Charles Popper, M.D.

Psychobiology of Bulimia (#10)
Edited by James I. Hudson, M.D., and Harrison G. Pope, Jr., M.D.

Cerebral Hemisphere Function in Depression (#11)
Edited by Marcel Kinsbourne, M.D.

Eating Behavior in Eating Disorders (#12)
Edited by B. Timothy Walsh, M.D.

Tardive Dyskinesia: Biological Mechanisms and Clinical Aspects (#13)
Edited by Marion E. Wolf, M.D., and Aron D. Mosnaim, Ph.D.

Current Approaches to the Prediction of Violence (#14)
Edited by David A. Brizer, M.D., and Martha L. Crowner, M.D.

Treatment of Tricyclic-Resistant Depression (#15)
Edited by Irl L. Extein, M.D.

Depressive Disorders and Immunity (#16)
Edited by Andrew H. Miller, M.D.

Depression and Families: Impact and Treatment (#17)
Edited by Gabor I. Keitner, M.D.

Depression in Schizophrenia (#18)
Edited by Lynn E. DeLisi, M.D.

Biological Assessment and Treatment of Posttraumatic Stress Disorder (#19)
Edited by Earl L. Giller, Jr., M.D., Ph.D.

Personality Disorders: New Perspectives on Diagnostic Validity (#20)
Edited by John M. Oldham, M.D.

Serotonin in Major Psychiatric Disorders (#21)
Edited by Emil F. Coccaro, M.D., and Dennis L. Murphy, M.D.

Amino Acids in Psychiatric Disease (#22)
Edited by Mary Ann Richardson, Ph.D.

Family Environment and Borderline Personality Disorder (#23)
Edited by Paul Skevington Links, M.D.

Biological Rhythms, Mood Disorders, Light Therapy, and the Pineal Gland (#24)
Edited by Mohammad Shafii, M.D.,
and Sharon Lee Shafii, R.N., B.S.N.

Treatment Strategies for Refractory Depression (#25)
Edited by Steven P. Roose, M.D.,
and Alexander H. Glassman, M.D.

Combination Pharmacotherapy and Psychotherapy for Depression (#26)
Edited by Donna Manning, M.D., and Allen J. Frances, M.D.

The Neuroleptic Nonresponsive Patient: Characterization and Treatment (#27)
Edited by Burt Angrist, M.D., and S. Charles Schulz, M.D.

Negative Schizophrenic Symptoms: Pathophysiology and Clinical Implications (#28)
Edited by John F. Greden, M.D., and Rajiv Tandon, M.D.

Neuropeptides and Psychiatric Disorders (#29)
Edited by Charles B. Nemeroff, M.D., Ph.D.

Central Nervous System Peptide Mechanisms in Stress and Depression (#30)
Edited by S. Craig Risch, M.D.

Current Concepts of Somatization: Research and Clinical Perspectives (#31)
Edited by Laurence J. Kirmayer, M.D., F.R.C.P.C.,
and James M. Robbins, Ph.D.

Mental Retardation: Developing Pharmacotherapies (#32)
Edited by John J. Ratey, M.D.

Positron-Emission Tomography in Schizophrenia Research (#33)
Edited by Nora D. Volkow, M.D., and Alfred P. Wolf, Ph.D.

Brain Imaging in Affective Disorders (#34)
Edited by Peter Hauser, M.D.

Psychoimmunology Update (#35)
Edited by Jack M. Gorman, M.D., and Robert M. Kertzner, M.D.

Biology of Anxiety Disorders (#36)
Edited by Rudolf Hoehn-Saric, M.D.,
and Daniel R. McLeod, Ph.D.

Multiple Sclerosis: A Neuropsychiatric Disorder (#37)
Edited by Uriel Halbreich, M.D.

The Clinical Science of Electroconvulsive Therapy (#38)
C. Edward Coffey, M.D.

Psychopharmacology and Psychobiology of Ethnicity (#39)
Edited by Keh-Ming Lin, M.D., M.P.H., Russell E. Poland, Ph.D., and Gayle Nakasaki, M.S.W.

Chronic Fatigue and Related Immune Deficiency Syndromes (#40)
Edited by Paul J. Goodnick, M.D., and Nancy G. Klimas, M.D.

Foreword

Psychopharmacology, psychobiology, and ethnicity are all heavy words, each with its own dictionary definition. Their combined use in a book title indicates a struggle—a medical struggle to break new ground. They also bring up a major question: When assessing and treating psychiatric illness, how important is it to keep in mind that the patient is a descendant of people with a distinct biological and cultural background, in addition to being an individual?

Until several decades ago, individuality was often ignored by the medical profession; treatment tended to be standardized, disregarding interindividual differences in responses. Then, in the 1950s and 1960s, came the discovery of enzyme induction and the realization that intake of certain foods or drugs could adaptively modify drug metabolism and thereby drug response. Concurrently, there was the rise of pharmacogenetics and an increased understanding of inborn differences in drug metabolism and/or drug response. More recently we have begun to realize how both adaptive and genetic forces may cause pharmacological distinctions between human populations who were in the past, or are currently, separated by distances or other geographical barriers.

This book provides a unique overview of the cases and the causes of differences between ethnically defined populations as they respond to psychoactive drugs. Biochemical distinctions may result in dissimilar benefits of drug treatment, as well as variations in drug toxicity or addiction liabilities. However, much of this important new knowledge is still fragmentary. We often do not know which drugs are and which are not affected by a given enzyme variant. If affected, how important is this clinically? How frequent are certain metabolic deficiencies in particular populations? Should recommendations for dosage of a drug be deliberately altered in some populations? Many questions remain to be answered that will require collective efforts for a long time to come.

While providing some initial answers to these important questions, this book also will give the reader a taste of some of the research that is currently being pursued in different laboratories. In addition, the existence of this book illustrates that interethnic variation in drug response and the interpretation of "biological markers" is becoming a recognized area worthy of a combination of efforts. This is most clearly demonstrated by the recent establishment of the Research Center on the Psychobiology of Ethnicity, at the Harbor-UCLA Medical Center, Research and Education Institute, Inc., in Torrance, California, which has been made possible with support by the National Institute of Mental Health: without this center, this book would not have been written. Another equally encouraging sign is the founding of the Pacific Rim Association for Clinical Pharmacogenetics, a high-caliber academic organization with the aim to stimulate interethnic research. Several members of this Association are authors of chapters in this book. With a concerted effort of scientists and clinicians associated with these and other prominent organizations, there is reason to believe that the field will progress in an accelerated fashion, and cross-ethnic psychiatric assessment and care can be done in an increasingly more informed and rational way.

Werner Kalow, M.D., F.R.S.C.

Section I

Introduction and Overview

Chapter 1

Introduction: Psychopharmacology, Psychobiology, and Ethnicity

Keh-Ming Lin, M.D., M.P.H., Russell E. Poland, Ph.D., and Gayle Nakasaki, M.S.W.

In this book, contributors review and summarize our current knowledge of ethnic differences and similarities in response to psychotropic drugs as well as in the interpretation of neurobiological correlates ("biological markers") of psychiatric disorders. Capitalizing on recent advances in biological and cross-cultural research methodologies, progress in this area has been remarkable. Increasingly sophisticated technologies—especially in the fields of pharmacokinetics, molecular biology, and brain imaging—have become available for cross-ethnic psychopharmacologic and psychopathological research. Consequently, many of the findings contained in the following chapters are intriguing, thought-provoking, and clinically relevant. However, since this is still a very new area of scientific investigation, many important issues still await further clarification. Although new technologies make it possible to more precisely and quantitatively examine some of the existing questions (e.g., are there biologically determined differences in response to certain psychotropics among ethnic groups?), they often will raise more fundamental questions (e.g., what is the main cause of such differences?). These questions can only be answered with the aid of newer advances for the assessment of the mechanisms responsible for the regulation of drug metabolism and the effects of medications on the

Supported in part by Research Center on the Psychobiology of Ethnicity MH47193 (Drs. Lin, Poland, and Silver) and National Institute of Mental Health Research Scientist Development Award MH00534 (Dr. Poland).

central nervous system (e.g., genotyping; study of drug-receptor interactions by brain imaging).

Despite the apparent complexity of the issues involved, the continuing progress in this area is important for several major reasons that will be elaborated on in the following section.

SIGNIFICANCE OF ETHNICITY IN PSYCHOPHARMACOLOGICAL AND PSYCHOBIOLOGICAL RESEARCH

First, an understanding of ethnicity and its psychopharmacological and psychobiological correlates is vital for ensuring quality psychiatric care for the ethnic minority populations in this country. Psychopharmacotherapy is essential for the treatment of the majority of severely mentally ill people, and advances in the search for biological markers are likely to revolutionize the practice of psychiatric diagnosis and care in the coming decade (Freedman 1987; Schuckit 1988). With rare exceptions, research in these vitally important areas has neglected ethnic minority populations (Lawson 1986). Such neglect is increasingly more problematic because of the phenomenal ongoing population shifts that have been taking place in recent decades. According to the 1990 U.S. census report, "non-Anglos" already represent 25% of the total population (including 12% African-Americans, 9% Hispanic-Americans, 3% Asian-Americans, and 1% American Indians). Because this trend of rapid growth in the minority sectors will likely continue (Spencer 1986), the majority of American psychiatrists will be expected to routinely provide care for a large number of patients of divergent ethnic/cultural backgrounds, and clinicians will no longer be able to neglect ethnic and cultural factors in the clinical care of their patients.

In addition, 80% of all people live outside North America and Western Europe (Kleinman 1988; Mezzich et al. 1992; United Nations 1988). Unlike other systems of psychiatric theories and practices originally developed in Western countries, which have thus far achieved very limited successes in non-Western countries, the introduction of psychopharmacotherapy and biological psychiatry has encountered little if any resistance in cross-cultural and cross-national dissemination (Lin and Poland 1989; Lin et al. 1986). However, as most of the original research in these fields has been conducted on Western populations, an uncritical acceptance of the results derived from such research by non-Western clinicians may be problematic. A greater understanding of cross-ethnic differences and similarities in the efficacy of biological treatment methods and the application and interpretation of biological markers would ensure the proper transfer of these therapeutic and assessment technologies across cultural and national boundaries (Lin et al. 1990). In addition, information regarding the patterns and mechanisms of ethnic differences in drug responses will also enable governments and pharmaceutical companies to more appropriately evaluate and make scientifically sound decisions on the relevance and utility of data already collected and analyzed in other countries. This will help to avoid duplication of effort and facilitate the development and introduction of new drugs for clinical use (Kalow 1990).

Because factors that may be responsible for ethnic differences in the response to treatment and interpretation of biological markers are often identical to those responsible for interindividual variations (Clark et al. 1988; Kalow et al. 1986; Lin et al. 1986, 1990), progress in the former is likely to lead to a better understanding in the latter, and vice versa. Thus, cross-ethnic research is likely to contribute to better psychiatric care for nonminority patients as well.

Finally, cross-ethnic studies are essential for differentiating between and among various psychiatric practices or theories that are culturally specific (i.e., only applicable to a particular ethnic or cultural group) and those that are "universal." In this sense, the significance of research aimed at clarifying cross-ethnic differences and similarities is not limited only to its practical application, but also has important theoretical implications (Kleinman 1988; Sartorius and Jablensky 1976). If particular biological abnormalities and responses are comparable in all ethnic groups, then this would strongly support the existence of comparable (universal) pathophysiologic underpinnings for the disease or disorder. In contrast, if an ethnic group does not manifest the "abnormal" biological parameter purported to be associated with a particular psychiatric disorder, then the pathophysiologic relevance of the biological marker would require rethinking. "Cross-ethnic" validation thus represents a powerful tool for psychiatric research, and results of such studies could prove extremely helpful in guiding future directions of scientific investigations.

ETHNICITY, RACE, AND CULTURE

Because terms such as "ethnicity," "race," and "culture" will be used repeatedly throughout this book, it appears important that their definitions and relationship with each other be clarified at the outset. Unfortunately, this is not as easy as it seems. Like many basic concepts, these seemingly simple and widely utilized terms become far more elusive and ambiguous upon closer scrutiny. Traditionally, "race" has been used to denote groupings that are biologically (and presumably genetically) determined, whereas "culture" represents attributes that are learned and passed down from generation to generation. Characteristics that are said to be racially determined (e.g., skin color) are supposed to be inherited and immutable, whereas culturally determined traits (e.g., ritualistically or medically performed circumcision; foot-binding, which was practiced in China until several decades ago; and the sloping of the forehead of pre-Columbian Mayans, which was produced by constant pressuring on children's heads during early childhood) are shaped by traditions and customs. Theoretically, it is possible to have groups with similar racial but different cultural backgrounds, and vice versa.

In reality, the use of the term "race" has been problematic. This is so not only because the concept has heavy political connotations and has been associated with large-scale injustice and atrocities throughout human history, but even more importantly, because it conveys a false sense of distinctiveness among different "racial" groups as currently defined and implies the existence of biological basis and accuracy of such classification systems (Cooper and David 1986; Cruickshank and Beevers 1989). Because of this, the United Nations has discouraged the continuing use of the term "race" and has recommended replacing it with "ethnic group" (Montagu 1960; Polednak 1989). Although harder to define, "ethnic group" and, by extension, "ethnicity," have become the terms preferred by most researchers in the field (Sue

1991). These terms connote groups of individuals who typically share ancestral and cultural commonalities as well as a sense of shared identity (McGoldrick et al. 1982; Shibutani and Kwan 1965). Thus, the term "ethnicity" and its derivative(s) will be used throughout this book, and the term "race" will be avoided unless in the context of a quotation. The term "culture" will be used only when the context of the discussion involves purely nonbiological issues (e.g., influences of childrearing practices; significance of belief systems).

AN OUTLINE OF THIS BOOK

This book is divided into three sections. Section I, Introduction and Overview, contains three chapters. In Chapter 2, the authors systematically review the literature on ethnic influences on drug responses and the interpretation and significance of biological parameters. Unlike the rest of the book, this chapter focuses primarily on findings derived from fields other than psychiatry. One of the purposes of such a review is to provide a broader perspective and context for subsequent chapters. In Chapter 3, the authors review nonpharmacological issues, such as compliance and placebo effects, in the context of culture.

Section II, Ethnicity and Psychopharmacology, contains seven chapters. The first three chapters extensively review the existing literature on the relationship between ethnicity and tricyclic antidepressants (Chapter 4), benzodiazepines (Chapter 5), and lithium (Chapter 6). These reviews summarize reports indicating ethnic differences and similarities in responding to these categories of psychotropics and discuss possible mechanisms underlying ethnic variations in responses and future research directions. The next three chapters examine ethnic factors in neuroleptic responses from different angles. In Chapter 7, the mechanism(s) that could be responsible for ethnic differences in response to haloperidol are discussed. The chapter also describes new methods for directly measuring the enzymes responsible for converting haloperidol to reduced haloperidol (haloperidol reductase). In Chapter 8, the authors report findings of a trans-Pacific, multiethnic comparison of the steady-state concentrations of haloperidol. They demonstrate substantial variations across four ethnic groups in their kinetic profiles and dose requirements. They further report that such differences could be partially explained by ethnic variation in the ratio between haloperidol and a major metabolite, reduced haloperidol. This is followed by a comprehensive review of studies comparing the rates and severity of tardive dyskinesia in different ethnic communities (Chapter 9). Finally, in Chapter 10, the author provides a concise review of the very rich and still rapidly growing literature on ethnic differences in the "flushing response" and intolerance to alcohol, biochemical and genetic bases for such intolerance, and its relationship to the propensity of developing alcoholism.

Section III, Ethnicity and Psychobiology, includes three chapters. In Chapter 11, the authors provide an overview of the mostly sporadic reports of ethnic differences in various biological measurements and bioneurological correlates, both in psychiatric patients and control subjects. This is followed by a discussion of the use of the stress reactivity research model to study depression in different ethnic settings (Chapter 12). In Chapter 13, the authors discuss ethnic and cultural issues in the evaluation and care of patients with dementia.

Because these are all fairly new areas of research, many important pieces of this puzzle are still missing, making the interpretation of study results difficult at times. However, as will be seen, despite obvious limitations, progress in the field as a whole has been truly remarkable in the past decade. We believe that the material presented in this book will serve to provide a state-of-the-art summary and synthesis of our knowledge and understanding of various issues being discussed. At the same time, we also hope that this book will substantially spur research in cross-cultural psychobiology.

REFERENCES

Clark WG, Brater DG, Johnson AR (eds): Goth's Medical Pharmacology, 12th Edition. St. Louis, MO, CV Mosby, 1988

Cooper R, David R: The biological concept of race and its application to public health and epidemiology. J Health Polit Policy Law 11:97–116, 1986

Cruickshank JK, Beevers DG: Ethnic Factors in Health and Disease. London, Wright, 1989
Freedman DX: Strategies for research in biological psychiatry, in Psychopharmacology: The Third Generation of Progress. Edited by Meltzer HY. New York, Raven, 1987, pp 23–30
Kalow W: Pharmacogenetics: past and future. Life Sci 47:1385–1397, 1990
Kalow W, Goedde HW, Agarwal DP (eds): Ethnic Differences in Reactions to Drugs and Xenobiotics. New York, Alan R Liss, 1986
Kleinman AM: Rethinking Psychiatry. New York, Free Press, 1988
Lawson WB: Racial and ethnic factors in psychiatric research. Hosp Community Psychiatry 37:50–54, 1986
Lin KM, Poland RE: Pharmacotherapy of Asian psychiatric patients. Psychiatric Annals 19:659–663, 1989
Lin KM, Poland RE, Lesser IM: Ethnicity and psychopharmacology. Cult Med Psychiatry 10:151–165, 1986
Lin KM, Poland RE, Chien CP: Ethnicity and psychopharmacology: recent findings and future research directions, in Family, Culture and Psychobiology. Edited by Dorel E. New York, Legas, 1990, pp 111–131
McGoldrick M, Pearce JK, Giordano J: Ethnicity and Family Therapy. New York, Guilford, 1982
Mezzich JE, Fabrega H, Kleinman A: Cultural validity and DSM-IV. J Nerv Ment Dis 180:1, 1992
Montagu AMF: Manual of Physical Anthropology. Springfield, IL, Charles C Thomas, 1960
Polednak AP: Racial and Ethnic Differences in Disease. New York, Oxford University Press, 1989
Sartorius N, Jablensky A: Transcultural studies of schizophrenia. WHO Chronicle 30:481–485, 1976
Schuckit MA: Trait and state markers of a predisposition to psychopathology, in Psychiatry, Vol 3, Chapter 53. Edited by Michels R. Philadelphia, PA, JB Lippincott, 1988, pp 1–19
Shibutani T, Kwan KM: Ethnic stratification. New York, Macmillan, 1965
Spencer G: Projections of the Hispanic populations: 1983 to 2080. Washington, DC, U.S. Department of Commerce, Bureau of the Census, 1986
Sue S: Ethnicity and culture in psychological research and practice, in Psychological Perspectives on Human Diversity in America. Edited by Goodchilds JD. Washington, DC, American Psychological Association, 1991, pp 47–86
United Nations: 1986 Demographic Yearbook. New York, Department of International Economic and Social Affairs, Statistical Office, United Nations, 1988

Chapter 2

Overview: The Interface Between Psychobiology and Ethnicity

Keh-Ming Lin, M.D., M.P.H., Russell E. Poland, Ph.D., and Barbara Silver, M.D.

In the field of psychiatry, there has been a widespread dichotomy that separates psychobiological research and studies aimed at clarifying how ethnic and cultural factors influence psychopathology and treatment response (Adebimpe 1980; Canino et al. 1991; Lawson 1986). Consciously or unconsciously, researchers whose primary interests are in the area of biological psychiatry often assume biological processes and phenomena to be "universal," and thus perhaps "color-blind." In contrast, social scientists and cross-cultural psychiatrists have tended to focus their attention primarily on how social forces and cultural traditions impinge on human behavior. Thus, the area between biological and cultural psychiatry has remained a borderland, simultaneously neglected by both disciplines.

Interestingly, while the issues concerning the interface between biology and ethnicity have remained peripheral to psychiatry, they have increasingly become the focus of intensive and systematic investigations in other branches of health sciences, such as pharmacology (Agarwal and Goedde 1990; Kalow 1989, 1990, 1991; Kalow et al. 1986; Weber 1987) and medical genetics (Cruickshank and Beevers 1989; Goodman 1979; Polednak 1989; Williams 1975). Some of these developments will be briefly reviewed here—not only because they are highly relevant to the

Supported in part by Research Center on the Psychobiology of Ethnicity MH47193 (Drs. Lin, Poland, and Silver) and National Institute of Mental Health Research Scientist Development Award MH00534 (Dr. Poland).

topics of this book, but even more importantly, because they will help to provide a broader, more theoretically based context for the discussions in subsequent chapters.

ETHNICITY AND PHARMACOGENETICS

Dramatic ethnic differences in response to drugs contributed substantially to the development of modern pharmacogenetics as a scientific discipline (Kalow 1990, 1991; Nebert and Weber 1990). The frequent occurrence of "primaquine hemolysis" among African-American soldiers fighting in Southeast Asia during World War II (Kalow 1991), which was subsequently found to be caused by an inborn deficiency of glucose-6-phosphate dehydrogenase (Dern et al. 1955), helped to launch systematic efforts in the search of genetic control of pharmacologic responses (Kalow 1990, 1991). In the early 1950s, isoniazid was used all over the world for the treatment of tuberculosis. Observations of ethnic differences in side effect profiles (Weber 1987) led to the identification of genetically controlled slow versus rapid acetylation phenotypes of isoniazid. Acetylation status has subsequently been found not only to determine the metabolism of a large number of pharmacoactive agents, including some frequently prescribed psychotropics (Lin et al. 1991; Mendoza et al. 1991; see Table 2–1), but it also is a significant risk factor for the development of a number of malignant conditions (Weber 1987). At present, acetylation status and its relevance to health and diseases represents an active area of research (Weber 1987).

The discovery of atypical alcohol dehydrogenase in 1965 and the genetic basis of aldehyde dehydrogenase deficiency in 1979

Table 2–1. Drugs subject to acetylation

Acebutolol	Dapsone	Prizidilol
p-Aminobenzoic acid	Dipyrone	Procainamide
p-Aminosalicylic acid	Endralazine	Sulfadiazine
Aminoglutethimide	Hydralazine	Sulfamerazine
Amrinone	Isoniazid	Sulfamethazine
Caffeine	Nitrazepam	Sulfapyridine
Clonazepam	Phenelzine	

also have their roots in earlier observations of large cross-ethnic variations in response to alcohol and in the frequency of the "flushing response" (Agarwal and Goedde 1990; Yamamoto et al. 1988; Yoshida 1983; see also Chapter 10). Along with the recent developments in molecular biology, a large number of ethnically specific variants of these enzymes have been identified. These findings have provided background information crucial to the understanding of ethnic differences in ethanol metabolism. Even more importantly, they also point to possible future research directions, including the identification of the gene(s) that may be responsible for the development of alcoholism, and the study of the metabolism of endogenous neurotransmitters, some of which are biotransformed by these two enzyme systems (Agarwal and Goedde 1990; Agarwal et al. 1982). Some of these issues will be discussed further in Chapter 10.

Many pharmacologically active agents are relatively nonpolar and require two metabolic steps—functionalization and conjugation—to be rendered sufficiently water-soluble for excretion. Phase I of the process, involving the addition of a functional group into the substrate, is predominantly carried out by the cytochrome P_{450} isozymes (Clark et al. 1988; Shen and Lin 1990). These enzymes may be regarded as one of the most important defense systems that have evolved in animals through the millennia to protect themselves against potentially harmful xenobiotics that they are routinely exposed to in their habitat (Gonzalez and Nebert 1990; Jackson 1991), either from their diet (e.g., various substances present in the edible plants) or through other means (e.g., exposure to pollens). In order for a limited number of these enzymes to metabolize and detoxify countless foreign substances, they have to be sufficiently "nonselective" (i.e., each single P_{450} enzyme can metabolize multiple substrates that are often structurally dissimilar). It is also this same quality that makes it possible for the P_{450} isozymes to metabolize and "detoxify" modern chemotherapeutic agents that are mostly synthetic and thus not the original targets for these enzymes.

Similar to the other examples discussed above, two of the P_{450} isozymes—debrisoquine hydroxylase (CYP2D6) and mephenytoin hydroxylase ($CYP2C_{mp}$)—have been found to be polymorphic, meaning that the enzyme activities are bimodally distributed in any given population, whose members can be classified as extensive metabolizers (EMs) or poor metabolizers (PMs), accordingly (Eichelbaum and Gross 1990; Gonzalez 1989; Kalow 1991; Meyer et al. 1990; Wilkinson et al. 1989; Wood and Zhou 1991). Subsequent molecular genetic studies revealed that such differences in the enzyme activities are genetically controlled: the enzymes are defective in PMs because of mutations in the nucleic acid sequence in the DNA; consequently, alterations occur in its corresponding amino acid structure in the enzyme. Studies involving these two enzymes may be of particular significance for psychiatry, because they are responsible for the metabolism of many commonly used psychotropics (Table 2–2), including tricyclic antidepressants (Bertilsson and Aberg-Wistedt 1983; Bertilsson et al. 1980; Mellstrom et al. 1983; Skjelbo et al. 1991), neuroleptics (Dahl-Puustinen et al. 1989), benzodiazepines (Bertilsson et al. 1989b; Wilkinson et al. 1989), barbiturates (Kupfer and Preisig 1984), and propranolol (Shaheen et al. 1989; Ward et al. 1989). In addition, recent studies have reported that the PM phenotype of debrisoquine hydroxylase may be related to higher incidence of parkinsonism (Barbeau et al. 1985; Otton et al. 1983) and to unique personality traits (Bertilsson et al. 1989a), suggesting that the functional variation of this enzyme may not be limited only to the liver but may also be present in the brain.

Interestingly, substantial cross-ethnic differences in the frequency of PM phenotype also exist with these enzymes. As can

Table 2–2. Drugs subject to debrisoquine P_{450} enzyme metabolism

Alprenolol	Flecainide	Phenacetin
Amiflamine	Guanoxan	Phenformin
Amitryptiline	Imipramine	Propafenone
Bufuralol	Indoramin	Propranolol
Chlorpromazine	Methoxyphenamine	Sparteine
Clomipramine	Metiamide	Thioridazine
Codeine	Metoprolol	Timolol
Desipramine	Nortriptyline	Tomoxetine
Dextromethorphan	Perhexiline	
Encainide	Perphenazine	

be seen from Table 2–3, the frequency of PM of debrisoquine varies from less than 3% in Cuna Indians (Arias et al. 1988b; Jorge et al. 1990), Egyptians (Mahgoub et al. 1979), and Saudi Arabians (Islam et al. 1980), as well as several Asian subgroups including Chinese (Du and Lou 1990; Lee et al. 1988; Lou et al. 1987; Xu and Jiang 1990), Japanese (Horai et al. 1990; Ishizaki et al. 1987; Nakamura et al. 1985), Malayans (Lee et al. 1988), and Thais (Wanwimolruk et al. 1990), to 3%–10% in Caucasians and Hispanics in Europe and North America. A wider range of frequencies is found in black Africans, with 0%–8% of sub-Saharan Africans, 4% of Venda in South Africa, 1.9% of African-Americans, and 19% of Sans Bushmen being classified as PM. Data on PM of the O-methylation of dextromethorphan and oxidation of sparteine also are included in Table 2–3, as several studies indicated that these processes cosegregate with debrisoquine hydroxylation (Eichelbaum et al. 1982; Horai et al. 1990; Inaba et al. 1983). However, one study (Woolhouse et al. 1979) did not show a cosegregation of debrisoquine and sparteine hydroxylation in Ghanians.

Mephenytoin hydroxylation displays a discrete phenotypy from that of debrisoquine (Table 2–4). In contrast to findings that being a PM of debrisoquine is more frequent in Caucasians than Asians, PMs of mephenytoin are more prevalent in Asian populations, with approximately 20% of Japanese being classified as PMs (Horai et al. 1989; Jurima et al. 1985; Nakamura et al. 1985). Chinese from the People's Republic of China also demonstrate a high frequency of PMs (Horai et al. 1989), whereas Chinese in Canada display a much lower frequency (Jurima et al. 1985) similar to that of Caucasians (Drohse et al. 1989; Inaba et al. 1984; Jacqz et al. 1988; Jurima et al. 1985; Nakamura et al. 1985; Sanz et al. 1989; Wedlund et al. 1984).

Why do ethnic variations exist in so many vitally important enzymes? The phylogenetic basis of the glucose-6-dehydrogenase deficiency is understandable. This trait has been demonstrated to be associated with an increased resistance to malaria infection. Because the ancestors of most carriers of this trait originally came from malaria-infested areas, including central Africa, the selective survival value of such an attribute is self-evident (Kalow 1991). The evolutionary origins of the ethnic variation of

Table 2–3. Debrisoquine/dextromethorphan/sparteine oxidation

Authors	Country	Sample size	# (%) PM	Drug
Studies in Africans and African-Americans				
African-Americans				
Relling et al. 1991	U.S.	106	2 (1.9%)	DM
Sub-Saharan Africans				
Eichelbaum and Woodhouse 1985	Ghana	154	0 (0%)	SP
Iyun et al. 1986	Nigeria	137	0 (0%)	DB
Mbanefo et al. 1980	Nigeria	123	10 (8.1%)	DB
Woolhouse et al. 1979	Ghana	80	5 (6.3%)	DB
Sans Bushmen				
Sommers et al. 1988	S. Africa	96	18 (19%)	DB
Venda				
Sommers et al. 1989	S. Africa	98	4 (4.1%)	DB
Sommers et al. 1991	S. Africa	97	0 (0%)	SP
Studies in Central and South American Indians and Hispanics				
Cuna				
Arias et al. 1988b	Panama	170	0 (0%)	SP
Jorge et al. 1990	Panama	89	0 (0%)	DB
Hispanics				
Lam et al. 1991	U.S.	22	1 (4.5%)	DM
Ngawbe Guaymi				
Arias et al. 1988a	Panama	97	5 (5.2%)	SP
Studies in Asians				
Chinese				
Du and Lou 1990	China (Han)	140	2 (1.4%)	DB
Inaba et al. 1981	China	19	6 (32%)	DB
Kalow et al. 1980	Canada	13	4 (31%)	DB
Lee et al. 1988	Singapore	97	0 (0%)	DB
Lou et al. 1987	China	269	2 (.7%)	DB
Xu and Jiang 1990	China	220	3 (1.4%)	DB
Japanese				
Horai et al. 1990	Japan	55	1 (1.8%)	DB and SP
Ishizaki et al. 1987	Japan	84	2 (2.4%)	SP
Nakamura et al. 1985	Japan	100	0 (0%)	DB
Malayans				
Lee et al. 1988	Malaya	95	2 (2.1%)	DB
Thais				
Wanwimolruk et al. 1990	Thailand	173	2 (1.2%)	DB

Table 2–3. Debrisoquine/dextromethorphan/sparteine oxidation *(continued)*

Authors	Country	Sample size	# (%) PM	Drug
	Studies in Caucasians			
Arvela et al. 1988	Finland			DB
	(Finns)	155	5 (3.2%)	
	(Lapps)	70	6 (8.6%)	
Benitez et al. 1988	Spain	377	25 (6.6%)	DB
Drohse et al. 1989	Denmark	358	33 (9.2%)	SP
Inaba et al. 1983	Canada	80	6 (7.5%)	DB
Inaba et al. 1981	Canada	48	4 (8.3%)	SP
Inaba et al. 1984	Canada	83	6 (7.2%)	SP
Ishizaki et al. 1987	Germany	52	3 (5.8%)	SP
Jacqz et al. 1988	France	132	4 (3%)	DM
Kalow et al. 1980	Canada	38	2 (5%)	DB
Lam et al. 1991	U.S.	30	2 (6.7%)	DM
Leclercq et al. 1987	Belgium	167	12 (7.2%)	DB
Mahgoub et al. 1977 (race not stated)	Britain	94	3 (3.2%)	DB
Nakamura et al. 1985	U.S.	183	16 (8.7%)	DB
Peart et al. 1986	Australia	100	6 (6%)	DB
Price-Evans et al. 1980	Britain	258	23 (8.9%)	DB
Relling et al. 1991	U.S.	480	37 (7.7%)	DM
Sanz et al. 1989	Sweden	205	18 (8.9%)	DB
Schmid et al. 1985	Switzerland	268	23 (8.6%)	DM
Steiner et al. 1988	Sweden	757	41 (5.4%)	DB
Syvalahti et al. 1986	Finland	107	6 (5.6%)	DB
Szorady and Santa 1987	Hungary	100	8 (8%)	DB
Veronese and McLean 1991	Australia	152	13 (8.6%)	DB
Wedlund et al. 1984	U.S.	156	11 (7.0)	DB
	Studies in Egyptians			
Mahgoub et al. 1979	Egypt and Britain	72	1 (1.4%)	DB
	Studies in Saudi Arabians			
Islam et al. 1980	Saudi Arabia	102	1 (1%)	DB

Note. PM = poor metabolizer; DB = debrisoquine; DM = dextromethorphan; SP = sparteine.

the other enzymes are not as easily discernible. However, it is quite possible that they reflect differences in diet and other environmental factors to which the carriers' ancestors were exposed for hundreds of thousands of years. Ethnic groups originating from different parts of the world may vary widely in the ratio of heterozygotes to homozygotes that historically provided optimal survival advantage(s) secondary to improved prenatal or postna-

Table 2–4. Mephenytoin oxidation phenotypes

Authors	Country	Sample size	# (%) PMs
	Studies in East Indians		
Doshi et al. 1990	India	48	10 (20.8%)
	Studies in Central American Indians		
Inaba et al. 1988	Panama	90	0 (0%)
	Studies in Asians		
Chinese			
Horai et al. 1989	China	98	7 (17.4%)
Jurima et al. 1985	Canada	39	2 (5%)
Japanese			
Horai et al. 1989	Japan	200	45 (22%)
Jurima et al. 1985	Canada	31	7 (23%)
Nakamura et al. 1985	Japan	100	18 (18%)
	Studies in Caucasians		
Altieri and Kirshner 1991	U.S.	123	5 (4.1%)
Drohse et al. 1989	Denmark	358	9 (2.5%)
Inaba et al. 1984	Canada	83	2 (2.4%)
Jacqz et al. 1988	France	132	8 (6%)
Jurima et al. 1985	Canada	118	5 (4.2%)
Kupfer and Preisig 1984	Switzerland		(5%)
Lam et al. 1991	U.S.	30	2 (6.7%)
Nakamura et al. 1985	U.S.	183	5 (2.7%)
Sanz et al. 1989	Sweden	253	7 (2.8%)
Wedlund et al. 1984	U.S.	156	4 (2.6%)
	Studies in Hispanics		
Lam et al. 1991	U.S.	22	1 (4.8%)
	Studies in African-Americans		
Perel et al. 1991	U.S.	27	5 (18.5%)

Note. PM = poor metabolizer.

tal development in response to dietary selective pressure (Gonzalez and Nebert 1990).

ETHNICITY AND ENVIRONMENTAL INFLUENCES ON DRUG METABOLISM

In addition to genetic control, the activity of the cytochrome P_{450} enzymes can also be quite sensitive to environmental changes, including exposure to different diets, environmental toxins, and other drugs. This is also to be expected. To be effective, this important "defensive" enzyme system needs to be able to respond rapidly to changes in the environment. The role of the cytochrome P_{450}s in the induction and inhibition of the metabolism of various drugs, including psychotropics, has been reviewed in detail elsewhere (Murray and Reidy 1990) and will not be repeated here. Not as well known is the fact that diet often also influences the rate of metabolism of various drugs (Clark et al. 1988) and thus might also contribute to the observed ethnic differences in drug response.

For example, Branch and colleagues (1978) compared the rate of the biotransformation of antipyrine and found a significantly longer antipyrine half-life among Sudanese living in their home villages as compared to Sudanese living in Britain or to Caucasian Britons. The latter two groups metabolized antipyrine at similar rates, suggesting that environmental factors such as diet were responsible for the pharmacokinetic differences. Similar findings were reported in subsequent studies involving Asian Indians living in India, Asian Indian immigrants living in Britain, and Caucasian Britons (Dollery et al. 1979; Fraser et al. 1979). A follow-up study (Desai et al. 1980) found that among the immigrants, those who retained their dietary habits as lactovegetarians behaved similarly to those living in their home country, whereas the pharmacokinetic profiles of those who became meat eaters were indistinguishable from those of the Caucasian Britons.

As mentioned previously, recent studies involving debrisoquine have demonstrated that the frequency of PMs is much higher (6%–7%) in Caucasians than in Chinese (less than 1%). However, the average activity of the enzyme in the Chinese EMs is much lower than that of the Caucasian EMs (Kalow 1991). Although a genetic explanation of this apparently puzzling finding has been reported (Yue et al. 1989), the effect of environmental factors, such as dietary differences, could not yet be ruled out. Further, a recent study has demonstrated that the mean enzyme activities of mephenytoin hydroxylase in Chinese EMs are also significantly lower than those in Japanese EMs (Horai et al. 1989). These findings further strengthen the likelihood of environmental factors being important contributors to the ethnic differences in enzyme activities.

ETHNICITY AND PLASMA PROTEIN BINDING

Another consequence of the lipophilicity of most psychotropics is that they have to rely on plasma proteins for their transportation (Reidenberg and Erill 1986). Although various proteins as well as cells in the blood provide binding sites for psychotropics and other drugs, and thus function as carriers for these pharmacoactive agents, two categories of plasma proteins—$alpha_1$ acid glycoproteins (Baumann et al. 1988; Kremer et al. 1988) and albumins (Kragh-Hansen 1981)—are generally regarded as most important. Variations in the concentration of these drug-binding proteins in the plasma can significantly influence the effect of the drug by changing the free fraction and thus the amount of the unbound (free) drug concentrations in the plasma (DeLeve and Piafsky 1981; Levy and Moreland 1984; Routledge 1986). Because only the free (unbound) fraction of the drugs is usually pharmacologically active and capable of crossing the blood-brain barrier, changes in the concentrations of drug-binding proteins may have profound clinical significance (Baumann and Eap 1991; Crabtree et al. 1991). Theoretically, ethnic differences in plasma protein binding could occur because of genetic and/or environmental factors. The structures of these plasma proteins are genetically determined and have been shown to vary across ethnic groups in several studies (Fukuma et al. 1990; Juneja et al. 1988; Umetsu et al. 1988). It is at present unclear whether these structural differences could lead to differences in their drug-binding capacities. Thus far, very few cross-ethnic studies (Lin et al. 1991) of plasma protein binding have been conducted. Available studies have reported conflicting findings, indicating the need for more vigorous and systematic research in this area.

ETHNICITY AND PHARMACODYNAMICS

Ethnic differences in the pupillary responses to topical mydriatics were first reported in 1927 (Chen and Poth 1927). Since then, "impaired" mydriasis has been repeatedly observed in blacks and Asians following standard doses of epinephrine, cocaine, and atropine (Angenent and Koelle 1953; Garde et al. 1978; Scott 1945). This reduction in the mydriatic effect appears to be correlated with the degree of pigmentation of the irises and is not seen among albino black Africans, suggesting that this difference is not pharmacokinetically mediated. A recent study further demonstrated that blacks were also significantly less responsive to intramuscular atropine and scopolamine than Caucasians (Garde et al. 1978).

Soon after their introduction into the market, beta-blockers such as propranolol frequently were found to be ineffective in treating black hypertensive patients (Moser and Lunn 1981). In contrast, the doses of propranolol required for the effective treatment of hypertension were substantially smaller in Asians as compared to Caucasians (Zhou et al. 1989). Subsequent studies objectively demonstrated that the effects of propranolol on blood pressure and heart rate are most prominent in Asians and least apparent in black Africans and African-Americans, with Caucasians falling in between (Dimsdale et al. 1988; Johnson et al. 1992). These differences could not be explained by pharmacokinetic factors (Rutledge et al. 1989; Zhou et al. 1989). At the same time, several studies (Rutledge et al. 1989; Stein et al. 1990; Venter et al. 1985) have demonstrated that black Africans and African-Americans had significantly higher basal levels of lymphocytic cyclic AMP (cAMP) and greater cAMP response to the stimulatory effects of isoprenaline, indicating a higher degree of beta2-adrenoceptor activity in blacks. These studies together provided support to the concept that differences in the sensitivity of adreonceptors may be the major cause for the differential effects of propranolol and other beta-blockers in various ethnic groups (Kalow 1989).

Observations of the ethnic differences in therapeutic concentrations of various psychotropics (Chang et al. 1984, 1985; Hu et al. 1983; Takahashi 1979; Yamashita and Asano 1979; Yang 1985) and their neurohormonal effects (Lin et al. 1988) have led to speculation of the existence of ethnic differences in pharmacodynamics of these drugs. Some of these findings will be reviewed in the chapters on tricyclics and lithium in this book.

Psychotropics exert their effects by directly or indirectly interacting with brain receptors. In contrast to the rapid proliferations of findings of polymorphism and ethnic differences in genes controlling the enzymes responsible for drug metabolism, very little has been known about ethnic variations in the structure and functions of receptors. Kalow (1990) has argued that there are inherent constraints on the variability of the receptors. Because receptors are needed to respond to internal messengers (neurotransmitters), changes in the way they respond to stimulae will not only affect the effects of drugs but also their interaction with endogenous substrates. Such alterations are likely to lead to malfunctioning of the system. However, recent studies have demonstrated that the gene for dopamine D_2 receptor exists in two alleles (A1 and A2), whose relative prevalence varies significantly among different ethnic groups (Blum et al. 1990). Although the clinical relevance of the polymorphism of this receptor gene has not yet been clarified, it certainly points to a new direction of investigation that potentially could lead to a better understanding of the mechanisms responsible not only for ethnic differences in pharmacodynamics as indicated previously, but also to a greater understanding of psychopharmacologic processes in general.

ETHNICITY AND DISEASE SUSCEPTIBILITY

The culture/biology dichotomy, as mentioned earlier, has been a prevailing assumption that often is accepted uncritically by psychiatric researchers and clinicians. Rooted in the centuries-old philosophical debate over the relative importance of nature versus nurture in determining human behavior (Honigmann 1976), what appears to be cross-culturally similar or universal is typically regarded as the product of nature and assumed to be *biolog-*

ically determined. In this age of "biological psychiatry," the exponential growth in our knowledge of neurobiological processes thought to be potential substrates of various psychiatric syndromes has led to a widespread assumption that, because these conditions and their neurobiological correlates are (presumably) biologically determined, they should be universal. They are thus not expected to vary significantly across cultural and ethnic lines.

However, in other branches of medicine, where the etiology and pathophysiology of diseases have been much better defined and demarcated, remarkable cross-ethnic variations in prevalence and pathogenesis have typically been the rule rather than the exception (Cruickshank and Beevers 1989; Goodman 1979; Polednak 1989; Williams 1975). These include not only genetic disorders such as sickle cell anemia among sub-Saharan black Africans and African-Americans, Tay-Sachs disease among Ashkenazi Jews, and thalassemia and glucose-6-phosphate dehydrogenase deficiency–related hemolytic anemia among people in Africa, Mediterranean countries, and Southeast Asia, but also common disorders including hypertension, cardiovascular diseases, metabolic disorders, and a variety of malignant conditions. Furthermore, even where these conditions are cross-ethnically similar in their prevalence and/or clinical manifestations, they often are divergent in their etiology, clinical course, and treatment responses. For example, hypertension in blacks is predominantly volume dependent rather than secondary to high renin activity and usually responds to diuretics instead of beta-blockers (Cruickshank and Beevers 1989; Moser and Lunn 1981; Sowers et al. 1988; Williams 1975; see also Chapter 12). Similarly, although liver cirrhosis is a common condition in both Caucasian and Asian populations, the etiology, pathohistological changes, and clinical courses are ethnic-specific. Although the majority of liver cirrhosis patients seeking treatment in Europe and North America have conditions that are alcohol-related, those seen in Asia are predominantly associated with hepatitis B virus infection (Polednak 1989; Sung and Chen 1978).

In psychiatry, various "functional" syndromes have been increasingly regarded as "primarily" biological in nature, and presumably cross-culturally similar (Jablensky and Sartorius 1975, 1988; Leff 1981). Remarkably in contrast to this trend, organic mental disorders—at present the only psychiatric diagnoses that have well-delineated biological etiology and neurobiological correlates—demonstrate substantial cross-ethnic differences in their prevalence and associated risk factors (see also Chapter 13). Confronted with this apparent contradiction, one might ask if the appearance of the "universality" of "functional" psychiatric disorders is simply deceptive. Remarkable advances notwithstanding, our current understanding of the neurobiological substrates of psychiatric conditions, such as schizophrenia and major depression, may be comparable to what internal medicine knew about pneumonia before the discovery of bacteria and viruses, or about liver cirrhosis before the findings of "fatty liver" and hepatitis B antigens.

Following these analogies, it would appear reasonable to argue that conditions such as schizophrenia look similar cross-culturally, because we do not yet have the appropriate tools to distinguish various subtypes that may have divergent neurobiological correlates and may distribute differently in groups of people with dissimilar genetic and environmental backgrounds (Crow 1980; Tsuang et al. 1990). In all fairness, the extrapolation of findings from organic mental disorders and other medical disorders to "functional" psychiatric disorders remains a hypothesis awaiting systematic examination. It is certainly possible (although not likely) that the genes that are associated with major psychiatric syndromes have been so closely linked to behavioral patterns or diatheses essential for human survival since prehistorical times (Sloman 1976) that they have to be fairly equally distributed among any population. However, unless proven otherwise, the possibility of ethnic differences in the neurobiological correlates of psychiatric syndromes deserves careful scientific scrutiny (see Chapter 11). Kleinman (1988) pointed out that the World Health Organization's cross-national studies of schizophrenia and depression appear to carry an institutional bias that emphasizes cross-cultural similarities and plays down differences. This could be expected in a profession seeking to demonstrate that its conditions are universal. But this bias may confuse the role of biology as a source of differences with the need to show that psychiatric conditions are found worldwide. Here then, culture is an influence in psychiatric research itself.

In addition, a completely different line of evidence also suggests that culture can and should have important influences on neurobiological processes. Childrearing practices and training, as well as a variety of other kinds of childhood experiences, are to a significant degree culturally patterned and often diverge substantially among different cultures (Caudill and Weinstein 1969; Tobin et al. 1989). It has long been argued that these experiences, as well as the cultural forces behind them, can play a key role in the development and maturation of an individual and influence the way the whole nervous system comes to be organized and how it functions (Fabrega 1979). These claims are largely compatible with recent findings in cell biology (Kandel 1989) and neurodevelopment (Hoffman and Dobscha 1989; Huttenlocher 1979; Innocenti 1981; Ivy and Killackey 1982; O'Leary et al. 1981). These studies have clearly demonstrated that learning produces lasting changes in neuronal architecture and alterations in gene expression. These changes are particularly evident throughout childhood and adolescence, during which time there is also an ongoing elimination of axonal collaterals (Hoffman and Dobscha 1989). This "axonal pruning" may also be influenced by life experiences and, thus, culture. As research continues to push forward in these new frontiers of neuroscience, the effect of learning and life experiences in general on the structure and function of the brain will become increasingly elucidated. It is expected that through these studies, the role of culture in shaping neurobiological processes will also become more clarified.

CONCLUDING REMARKS

Psychiatry is a branch of medicine. As such, the principle and methodology that have been developed in other fields of medicine to a large extent should also apply to psychiatric practice and research; psychopharmacology provides a good example. The pharmacokinetic and pharmacodynamic principles that apply to drugs and xenobiotics in general are equally applicable to psychotropic medications. However, to a large extent, psychopharmacological practices and research have not benefited from recent development in clinical pharmacology. Reflecting this deficiency in interdisciplinary communication and collaboration, until recently psychiatrists and clinical pharmacologists who have reported ethnic differences in drug responses have done so separately and in parallel to each other. Similarly, in the race toward identifying "biological markers," psychiatric researchers tend not to pay attention to the remarkable cross-ethnic variability that exists in the prevalence and significance of various biological data in other fields of medicine and to equate biology with universality. We hope that the material presented in this chapter will serve to provide a general context against which the findings more immediately relevant to the field of psychopharmacology and psychobiology can be appropriately evaluated and appreciated. By so doing, we also hope that this chapter will in a small way spur interdisciplinary cross-fertilization, which will further promote the advancement in research in cross-cultural psychopharmacology and psychobiology.

REFERENCES

Adebimpe VR: Psychopharmacological norms in Blacks and Whites. Am J Psychiatry 137:870–871, 1980

Agarwal DP, Goedde HW: Alcohol Metabolism, Alcohol Intolerance and Alcoholism. Berlin, Springer-Verlag, 1990

Agarwal DP, Hafer G, Harada S, et al: Studies on aldehyde dehydrogenase and aldehyde reductase in human brain, in Enzymology of Carbonyl Metabolism: Aldehyde Dehydrogenase and Aldo-keto Reductase. Edited by Weiner H, Flynn TG. New York, Alan R Liss, 1982, pp 319–328

Angenent WJ, Koelle GB: A possible enzymatic basis for the differential action of mydriatics on light and dark irides. J Physiol 119:102–117, 1953

Arias TD, Inaba T, Cooke RG, et al: A preliminary note on the transient polymorphic oxidation of sparteine in the Ngawbe Guaymi Amerindians: a case of genetic divergence with tentative phylogenetic time frame for the pathway. Clin Pharmacol Ther 44:343–352, 1988a

Arias TD, Jorge D, Lee MD, et al: The oxidative metabolism of sparteine in the Cuna Amerindians of Panama: absence of evidence for deficient metabolizers. Clin Pharmacol Ther 43:456–465, 1988b

Arvela P, Kirjarinta M, Kirjarinta M, et al: Polymorphism of debrisoquine hydroxylation among Finns and Lapps. Br J Clin Pharmacol 26:601–603, 1988

Barbeau A, Cloutier T, Roy M, et al: Ecogenetics of Parkinson's disease: 4-hydroxylation of debrisoquine. Lancet 2:1213–1215, 1985

Baumann P, Eap CB: Alpha1-acid Glycoprotein Genetics, Biochemistry, Physiological Functions, and Pharmacology. New York, Alan R Liss, 1988

Baumann P, Eap CB: S-12-19-02 plasma monitoring of antidepressants: clinical relevance of the pharmacogenetics of metabolism and of $_1$-acid glycoprotein binding. Biol Psychiatry 29:7S–199S, 1991

Benitez J, Llerena A, Cobaleda J: Debrisoquine oxidation polymorphism in a Spanish population. Clin Pharmacol Ther 44:74–77, 1988

Bertilsson L, Aberg-Wistedt A: The debrisoquine hydroxylation test predicts steady-state plasma levels of desipramine. Br J Clin Pharmacol 15:388–390, 1983

Bertilsson L, Eichelbaum M, Mellstrom B, et al: Nortriptyline and antipyrine clearance in relation to debrisoquine hydroxylation in man. Life Sci 27:1673–1677, 1980

Bertilsson L, Alm C, DeLas Carreras, et al: Debrisoquine hydroxylation polymorphism and personality. Lancet 1:555, 1989a

Bertilsson L, Henthorn TK, Sanz E, et al: Importance of genetic factors in the regulation of diazepam metabolism: relationship to S-mephenytoin, but not debrisoquine, hydroxylation phenotype. Clin Pharmacol Ther 45:348–355, 1989b

Blum K, Noble EP, Sheridan PJ, et al: Allelic association of human dopamine D2 receptor gene in alcoholism. JAMA 263:2055–2060, 1990

Branch RA, Salih SY, Homeida M: Racial differences in drug metabolizing ability: a study with antipyrine in the Sudan. Clin Pharmacol Ther 24:283–286, 1978

Canino I, Chou JCY, Christmas JJ, et al: Cross-cultural issues and treatments of psychiatric disorders. Am J Psychiatry 148:543–544, 1991

Caudill W, Weinstein H: Maternal care and infant behavior in Japan and America. Psychiatry 32:12–43, 1969

Chang SS, Pandey GN, Davis JM, et al: Racial differences in plasma and RBC lithium levels. Paper presented at the annual meeting of the American Psychiatric Association. Continuing Medical Education Syllabus and Scientific Proceedings, 239–240, 1984

Chang SS, Pandey GN, Yang YY, et al: Lithium pharmacokinetics: interracial comparison. Presented at the 138th Annual Meeting of the American Psychiatric Association, Dallas, Texas, May 19–24, 1985

Chen KK, Poth EJ: The racial difference of the mydriastic action of ephedrines, cocaine, and euphthalmine. Proc Soc Exper Biol Med 25:150–151, 1927

Clark WG, Brater DG, Johnson AR (eds): Goth's Medical Pharmacology, 12th Edition. St. Louis, MO, CV Mosby, 1988

Crabtree BL, Jann MW, Pitts WM: Alpha$_1$ acid glycoprotein levels in patients with schizophrenia: effect of treatment with haloperidol. Biol Psychiatry 29:43A–185A, 1991

Crow TJ: Molecular pathology of schizophrenia: more than one disease process. BMJ 280:66–68, 1980

Cruickshank JK, Beevers DG: Ethnic Factors in Health and Disease. London, Wright, 1989

Dahl-Puustinen ML, Liden A, Alm C, et al: Disposition of perphenazine is related to polymorphic debrisoquine hydroxylation in human beings. Clin Pharmacol Ther 46:78–81, 1989

DeLeve LD, Piafsky KM: Clinical significance of plasma binding of basic drugs. Trends Pharmacol Sci 2:283–284, 1981

Dern RJ, Beutler E, Alving AS: The hemolytic effect of primaquine: the natural course of the hemolytic anemia and the mechanism of its self-limited character. J Lab Clin Med 44:171–176, 1955

Desai NK, Sheth UK, Mucklow JC, et al: Antipyrine clearance in Indian villagers. Br J Clin Pharmacol 9:387–394, 1980

Dimsdale J, Ziegler M, Graham R: The effect of hypertension, sodium, and race on isoproterenol sensitivity. Clin Exp Hypertens [A] 10:747–756, 1988

Dollery CT, Fraser HS, Mucklow JC, et al: Contribution of environmental factors to variability in human drug metabolism. Drug Metab Rev 9:207–220, 1979

Doshi BS, Kulkarni RD, Chauhan BL, et al: Frequency of impaired mephenytoin 4-hydroxylation in an Indian population. Br J Clin Pharmacol 30:779–780, 1990

Drohse A, Bathum L, Brosen K, et al: Mephenytoin and sparteine oxidation: genetic polymorphism in Denmark. Br J Clin Pharmacol 27:620–625, 1989

Du YL, Lou YQ: Polymorphism of debrisoquine 4-hydroxylation and family studies of poor metabolizers in Chinese population. Acta Pharmacologica Sinica 11:7–10, 1990

Eichelbaum M, Gross AS: The genetic polymorphism of debrisoquine/sparteine—clinical aspects. Pharmacol Ther 46:377–394, 1990

Eichelbaum M, Woolhouse NM: Inter-ethnic difference in sparteine oxidation among Ghanians and Germans. Eur J Clin Pharmacol 28:79–83, 1985

Eichelbaum M, Bertilsson L, Sawe J, et al: Polymorphic oxidation of sparteine and debrisoquine: related pharmacogenetic entities. Clin Pharmacol Ther 31:184–186, 1982

Fabrega H: Neurobiology, culture, and behavior disturbances: an integrative review. J Nerv Ment Dis 167:8, 1979
Fraser HS, Mucklow JC, Bulpitt CJ, et al: Environmental factors affecting antipyrine metabolism in London factory and office workers. Br J Clin Pharmacol 7:237–243, 1979
Fukuma Y, Kashimura S, Umetsu K, et al: Genetic variation of alpha-2-HS-glycoprotein in the Kyushu district of Japan: description of three new rare variants. Hum Hered 40:49–51, 1990
Garde JF, Aston R, Endler GC, et al: Racial mydriatic response to belladonna premedication. Anesth Analg 57:572–576, 1978
Gonzalez FJ: The molecular biology of cytochrome P450s. Pharmacol Rev 40:243–288, 1989
Gonzalez FJ, Nebert DW: Evolution of the P450 gene superfamily: animal-plant "warfare," molecular drive and human genetic differences in drug oxidation. Trends Genet 6:182–186, 1990
Goodman RM: Genetic Disorders Among the Jewish People. Baltimore, MD, Johns Hopkins University Press, 1979
Hoffman RE, Dobscha SK: Cortical pruning and the development of schizophrenia: a computer model. Schizophr Bull 15:477–489, 1989
Honigmann JJ: The Development of Anthropological Ideas. Homewood, IL, Dorsey Press, 1976
Horai Y, Nakano M, Ishizaki T, et al: Metoprolol and mephenytoin oxidation polymorphisms in Far Eastern oriental subjects: Japanese versus mainland Chinese. Clin Pharmacol Ther 46:198–207, 1989
Horai Y, Taga J, Ishizaki T, Ishikawa K: Correlations among the metabolic ratios of three test probes (metoprolol, debrisoquine, sparteine) for genetically determined oxidation polymorphism in a Japanese population. Br J Clin Pharmacol 29:111–115, 1990
Hu WH, Lee CF, Yang YY, et al: Imipramine plasma levels and clinical response. Bulletin of Chinese Society of Neurology and Psychiatry 9:40–49, 1983
Huttenlocher PR: Synaptic density in human frontal cortex—developmental changes and the effects of aging. Brain Res 163:195–205, 1979
Inaba T, Otton SV, Kalow W: Debrisoquine hydroxylation capacity: problems of assessment in two populations. Clin Pharmacol Ther 29:218–223, 1981
Inaba T, Vinks A, Otton S, et al: Comparative pharmacogenetics of sparteine and debrisoquine. Clin Pharmacol Ther 33:391–399, 1983
Inaba T, Jurima M, Nakano M, et al: Mephenytoin and sparteine pharmacogenetics in Canadian-Caucasians. Clin Pharmacol Ther 36:670–676, 1984

Inaba T, Jorge LF, Arias TD: Mephenytoin hydroxylation in the Cuna Amerindians of Panama. Br J Clin Pharmacol 25:75–79, 1988

Innocenti GM: Growth and reshaping of axons in the establishment of visual cortical callosal connections. Science 212:824–827, 1981

Ishizaki T, Eichelbaum M, Horai Y, et al: Evidence for polymorphic oxidation of sparteine in Japanese subjects. Br J Clin Pharmacol 23:482–485, 1987

Islam SI, Idle JR, Smith RL: The polymorphic 4-hydroxylation of debrisoquine in a Saudi Arab population. Xenobiotica 10:819–825, 1980

Ivy GO, Killackey HP: Ontogenetic changes in the projections of neurocortical neurons. J Neurol Sci 6:735–743, 1982

Iyun AO, Lennard MS, Tucker GT, Woods HF: Metoprolol and debrisoquine metabolism in Nigerians: lack of evidence for polymorphic oxidation. Clin Pharmacol Ther 40:387–394, 1986

Jablensky A, Sartorius N: Culture and schizophrenia. Psychol Med 5:113–124, 1975

Jablensky A, Sartorius N: Is schizophrenia universal? Acta Psychiatr Scand Suppl 344:65–70, 1988

Jackson FLC: Secondary compounds in plants (Allelochemicals) as promoters of human biological variability. Annu Rev Anthropol 20:505–546, 1991

Jacqz E, Dulac H, Mathieu H: Phenotyping polymorphic drug metabolism in the French Caucasian population. Eur J Clin Pharmacol 35:167–171, 1988

Johnson JA, Burlew BS, Sullivan JM: Racial differences in blood pressure response to increased forearm vascular resistance. Clin Pharmacol Ther 51:141, 1992

Jorge LF, Arias TD, Inaba T, et al: Unimodal distribution of the metabolic ratio for debrisoquine in Cuna Amerindians of Panama. Br J Clin Pharmacol 30:281–285, 1990

Juneja RK, Weitkamp LR, Stratil A, et al: Further studies of the plasma 1 β-glycoprotein polymorphism: two new alleles and allele frequencies in Caucasians and in American Blacks. Hum Hered 38:267–272, 1988

Jurima M, Inaba T, Kodar D, Kalow W: Genetic polymorphism of Mephenytoin p(4′) hydroxylation: difference between Orientals and Caucasians. Br J Clin Pharmacol 19:43–47, 1985

Kalow W: Race and therapeutic drug response. N Engl J Med 320:588–589, 1989

Kalow W: Pharmacogenetics: past and future. Life Sci 47:1385–1397, 1990

Kalow W: Interethnic variation of drug metabolism. Trends Pharmacol Sci (reprint), Vol 12, March 1991

Kalow W, Otton SV, Kada D, et al: Ethnic differences in drug metabolism: debrisoquine 4-hydroxylation in Caucasians and Orientals. Can J Physiol Pharmacol 58:1142–1144, 1980
Kalow W, Goedde HW, Agarwal DP (eds): Ethnic Differences in Reactions to Drugs and Xenobiotics. New York, Alan R Liss, 1986
Kandel ER: Genes, nerve cells, and the remembrance of things past. Journal of Neuropsychiatry 1:103–125, 1989
Kleinman AM: Rethinking Psychiatry. New York, Free Press, 1988
Kragh-Hansen U: Molecular aspects of ligand binding to serum albumin. Pharmacol Rev 33:1, 1981
Kremer JMH, Wilting J, Janssen LHM: Drug binding to human alpha-1-acid glycoprotein in health and disease. Pharmacol Rev 40:1, 1988
Kupfer A, Preisig R: Pharmacogenetics of mephenytoin: a new drug hydroxylation polymorphism in man. Eur J Clin Pharmacol 26:753–759, 1984
Lam YWF, Casto DT, Dunn JF: Drug metabolizing capacity in Mexican Americans. Clin Pharmacol Ther 49:159, 1991
Lawson WB: Racial and ethnic factors in psychiatric research. Hosp Community Psychiatry 37:50–54, 1986
Leclercq V, Desager JP, van Nieuwenhuyze Y, et al: Prevalence of drug hydroxylator phenotypes in Belgium. Eur J Clin Pharmacol 33:439–440, 1987
Lee EJ, Nam YP, Hee GN: Oxidation phenotyping in Chinese and Malay populations. Clin Exp Pharmacol Physiol 15:889–891, 1988
Leff J: Psychiatry Around the Globe: A Transcultural View. New York, Marcel Dekker, 1981
Levy RH, Moreland TA: Rationale for monitoring free drug levels. Clin Pharmacokinet 9 (suppl 1):1–9, 1984
Lin KM, Lau JK, Smith R, et al: Comparison of alprazolam plasma levels and behavioral effects in normal Asian and Caucasian male volunteers. Psychopharmacology (Berlin) 96:365–369, 1988
Lin KM, Poland RE, Smith MW, et al: Pharmacokinetic and other related factors affecting psychotropic responses in Asians. Psychopharmacol Bull 27:427–439, 1991
Lou Y, Ying L, Bertilsson L, et al: Low frequency of slow debrisoquine hydroxylation in a native Chinese population. Clin Pharmacol 15:443–450, 1987
Mahgoub A, Idle JR, Dring LG, et al: Polymorphic hydroxylation of debrisoquine in man. Lancet 2:584–586, 1977
Mahgoub A, Idle JR, Smith RL: A population and familial study of the defective alicyclic hydroxylation of debrisoquine among Egyptians. Xenobiotica 9:51–56, 1979

Mbanefo C, Barbanunmi EA, Mahgoub A, et al: A study of the debrisoquine hydroxylation polymorphism in a Nigerian population. Xenobiotica 10:811–818, 1980

Mellstrom B, Bertilsson L, Lou YC, et al: Amitriptyline metabolism: relationship to polymorphic debrisoquine hydroxylation. Clin Pharmacol Ther 34:516–520, 1983

Mendoza R, Smith MW, Poland RE, et al: Ethnic psychopharmacology: the Hispanic and Native American perspective. Psychopharmacol Bull 27:449–461, 1991

Meyer UA, Zanger UM, Grant D, et al: Genetic polymorphisms of drug metabolism. Advances in Drug Research 19:197–241, 1990

Moser M, Lunn J: Comparative effects of pindolol and hydrochlorothiazide in Black hypertensive patients. Angiology 32:561–566, 1981

Murray M, Reidy GF: Selectivity in the inhibition of mammalian cytochromes P-450 by chemical agents. Pharmacol Rev 42:2, 1990

Nakamura K, Goto F, Ray WA, et al: Interethnic differences in genetic polymorphism of debrisoquine and mephenytoin hydroxylation between Japanese and Caucasian populations. Clin Pharmacol Ther 38:402–408, 1985

Nebert DW, Weber WW: Pharmacogenetics, in Principles of Drug Action. Edited by Pratt WB, Taylor P. New York, Churchill Livingstone, 1990, pp 469–531

O'Leary DDM, Stanfield BB, Cowan WM: Evidence that the early postnatal restrictions of the cells of origin of the callosal projection is due to the elimination of axonal collaterals rather than the death of neurons. Developmental Brain Research 1:607–617, 1981

Otton SV, Inaba T, Kalow W: Inhibition of sparteine oxidation in human liver by tricyclic antidepressants and other drugs. Life Sci 32:795–800, 1983

Peart GF, Boatagy J, Shenfield GM: Debrisoquine oxidation in an Australian population. Br J Clin Pharmacol 21:465–471, 1986

Perel JM, Altieri L, Kirshner M: S-mephenytoin 4-hydroxylation in older Americans. Clin Pharmacol Ther 49:159, 1991

Polednak AP: Racial and Ethnic Differences in Disease. New York, Oxford University Press, 1989

Price-Evans DA, Mahgoub A, Sloan TP, et al: A family and population study of the genetic polymorphism of debrisoquine oxidation in a white British population. J Med Genet 17:102–105, 1980

Reidenberg MM, Erill S (eds): Drug-Protein Binding. New York, Praeger, 1986

Relling MV, Cherrie J, Schell MJ, et al: Lower prevalence of debrisoquine oxidation poor metabolizer phenotype in the American Black versus White subjects. Clin Pharmacol Ther 50:308–313, 1991

Routledge PA: The plasma protein binding of basic drugs. Br J Clin Pharmacol 22:499–506, 1986
Rutledge DR, Steinberg MB, Cardozo L: Racial differences in drug response: isoproterenol effects on heart rate following intravenous metoprolol. J Clin Pharmacol Ther 45:380–386, 1989
Sanz EJ, Villen T, Alm C, et al: S-mephenytoin hydroxylation phenotypes in a Swedish population determined after coadministration with debrisoquine. Clin Pharmacol Ther 45:495–499, 1989
Schmid B, Bircher J, Preisig R, et al: Polymorphic dextromethorphan metabolism: co-segregation of oxidative O-demethylation with debrisoquine hydroxylation. Clin Pharmacol Ther 38:618–624, 1985
Scott JG: The eye of the West African Negro. Br J Ophthal 29:12–15, 1945
Shaheen O, Biollaz J, Koshakji RP, et al: Influence of debrisoquine phenotype on the inducibility of propranolol metabolism. Clin Pharmacol Ther 45:439–443, 1989
Shen WW, Lin KM: Cytochrome P-450 monooxygenases and interactions of psychotropic drugs. Int J Psychiatry Med 21:21–30, 1990
Skjelbo E, Brosen K, Hallas J, et al: The mephenytoin oxidation polymorphism is partially responsible for the N-demethylation of imipramine. Clin Pharmacol Ther 49:18–23, 1991
Sloman L: The role of neurosis in phylogenetic adaptation, with particular reference to early man. Am J Psychiatry 133:543–547, 1976
Sommers DK, Moncrieff J, Avenant J: Polymorphism of the 4-hydroxylation of debrisoquine in the San Bushmen of southern Africa. Hum Toxicol 7:273–278, 1988
Sommers DK, Moncrieff J, Avenant J: Non-correlation between debrisoquine and metoprolol polymorphism in the Venda. Hum Toxicol 8:365–368, 1989
Sommers DK, Moncrieff J, Avenant JC: Absence of polymorphism of sparteine oxidation in the South African Venda. Hum Exp Toxicol 10:175–180, 1991
Sowers Jr, Zemel MB, Zemel P, et al: Salt sensitivity in blacks: salt intake and natriuretic substances. Hypertension 12:485–490, 1988
Stein M, O'Malley K, Kilfeather S: Ethnic differences in cyclic AMP accumulation: effect on $alpha_2$, $beta_2$, and prostanoid receptor responses. Clin Pharmacol Ther 47:360–365, 1990
Steiner E, Bertilsson L, Sawe J, et al: Polymorphic debrisoquine hydroxylation in 757 Swedish subjects. Clin Pharmacol Ther 44:431–435, 1988
Sung JL, Chen DS: Clustering of different subtypes of hepatitis B surface antigen in families of patients with chronic liver diseases. Am J Gastroenterol 69:559–564, 1978

Syvalahti EKG, Lindberg R, Kallio J, et al: Inhibitory effects of neuroleptics on debrisoquine oxidation in man. Br J Clin Pharmacol 22:89–92, 1986

Szorady I, Santa A: Drug hydroxylator phenotype in Hungary. Eur J Clin Pharmacol 32:325, 1987

Takahashi R: Lithium treatment in affective disorders: therapeutic plasma level. Psychopharmacol Bull 15:32–35, 1979

Tobin JJ, Wu DYH, Davidson DH: Preschool in Three Cultures: Japan, China, and the United States. New Haven, CT, Yale University Press, 1989

Tsuang MT, Lyons MJ, Faraone SV: Heterogeneity of schizophrenia: conceptual models and analytic strategies. Br J Psychiatry 156:17–26, 1990

Umetsu K, Yuasa I, Nishimura H, et al: T: Genetic polymorphisms of orosomucoid and alpha-2-HS-glycoprotein in a Philippine population. Hum Hered 38:287–290, 1988

Venter CP, Daya S, Joubert PH, et al: Ethnic differences in human lymphocytic cyclic AMP production after isoprenaline stimulation and propranolol blockade. Br J Clin Pharmacol 19:187–190, 1985

Veronese ME, McLean S: Debrisoquine oxidation polymorphism in a Tasmanian population. Eur J Clin Pharmacol 40:529–532, 1991

Wanwimolruk S, Patamasucon P, Lee EJD: Evidence for the polymorphic oxidation of debrisoquine in the Thai population. Br J Clin Pharmacol 29:244–247, 1990

Ward SE, Walle T, Walle UK, et al: Propranolol's metabolism is determined by both mephenytoin and debrisoquin hydroxylase activities. Clin Pharmacol Ther 45:72–79, 1989

Weber WW: The Acetylator Genes and Drug Responses. New York, Oxford University Press, 1987

Wedlund PJ, Aslanian WS, McAllister CB, et al: Mephenytoin hydroxylation deficiency in Caucasians: frequency of a new oxidative drug metabolism polymorphism. Clin Pharmacol Ther 36:773–780, 1984

Wilkinson GR, Guengerich FP, Branch RA: Genetic polymorphism of S-mephenytoin hydroxylation. Pharmacol Ther 43:53–76, 1989

Williams RA: Textbook of Black-Related Diseases. New York, McGraw-Hill, 1975

Wood AJJ, Zhou HH: Ethnic differences in drug disposition and responsiveness. Clin Pharmacokinet 20:1–24, 1991

Woolhouse NM, Andoh B, Mahgoub A, et al: Debrisoquine hydroxylation polymorphism among Ghanians and Caucasians. Clin Pharmacol Ther 26:584–591, 1979

Xu XM, Jiang WD: Debrisoquine hydroxylation and sulfamethazine acetylation in a Chinese population. Acta Pharmacologica Sinica 11:387–388, 1990

Yamamoto J, Yeh EK, Le CK, et al: Alcohol abuse among Koreans and Taiwanese, in Cultural Influences and Drinking Patterns: A Focus in Hispanic and Japanese Populations (Research Monograph No 19). Edited by Towle LH, Harford TC. Rockville, MD, National Institute on Alcohol Abuse and Alcoholism, 1988

Yamashita I, Asano Y: Tricyclic antidepressants: therapeutic plasma level. Psychopharmacol Bull 15:40–41, 1979

Yang YY: Prophylactic efficacy of lithium and its effective plasma levels in Chinese bipolar patients. Acta Psychiatr Scand 71:171–175, 1985

Yoshida A: Differences in the isozymes involved in alcohol metabolism between Caucasians and Orientals, in Isozymes: Current Topics in Biological and Metabolic Research (Vol 8: Cellular Localization, Metabolism, and Physiology). Edited by Rattazzi MC, Scandelios JG, Whitt GS. New York, Alan R Liss, 1983, pp 245–261

Yue QY, Bertilsson L, Dahl-Puustinen ML, et al: Disassociation between debrisoquine hydroxylation phenotype and genotype among Chinese. Lancet 2:870, 1989

Zhou HH, Koshakji RP, Silberstein DJ, et al: Altered sensitivity to and clearance of propranolol in men of Chinese descent as compared with American whites. N Engl J Med 320:565–570, 1989

Chapter 3

"Nonbiological" Issues Affecting Psychopharmacotherapy: Cultural Considerations

**Michael Smith, M.D.,
Keh-Ming Lin, M.D., M.P.H.,
and Ricardo Mendoza, M.D.**

Although the significance of various "nonbiological" factors—such as compliance (Becker 1985; Becker and Maiman 1980) and placebo effects (White et al. 1985)—in affecting the outcome of psychopharmacotherapy is widely recognized, they have rarely been the focus of systematic research efforts. Consequently, our understanding of these extremely important issues remains rudimentary, fragmented, and not scientifically based. This is problematic because the effects of pharmacoactive agents, especially psychotropics, are not solely determined by their pharmacological properties. The prescription and use of medication is enmeshed in a process replete with social and symbolic meanings and implications—one involving constant interaction and communication (or miscommunication) between clinicians, patients, and, frequently, the significant others of those patients (Moerman 1979).

Because these "nonbiological" factors are strongly influenced by sociocultural forces, it is reasonable to believe that they should be responsible for at least some of the clinically observed ethnic differences in psychotropic responses. However, practically all of the major studies in cross-cultural psychopharmacology have

Supported in part by MH47355 (Dr. Lin) and Research Center on the Psychobiology of Ethnicity MH47193 (Drs. Lin and Mendoza).

focused on biological variables (e.g., pharmacokinetics, pharmacogenetics, and pharmacodynamics; see Chapters 1 and 2). Thus, perhaps somewhat paradoxically, at present we know relatively more about the biological rather than the sociocultural contributions involved in the differential response to psychotropic medications displayed by various ethnic groups (Lin et al. 1990: see also Chapters 4 through 10 in Section II). This notwithstanding, we believe that in a book such as this, cultural and "nonbiological" issues should not be neglected.

In this chapter, we will systematically survey these issues and discuss their relevance in cross-cultural settings. We will start with a general discussion of the importance of culturally held health beliefs. A commentary on other factors such as compliance, placebo effects, personality factors, effects of social support and stress, and diagnostic issues then follows. We hope the material presented here will be of use to clinicians providing psychopharmacotherapy to ethnic minority patients on a regular basis. In addition, we hope to stimulate interest in more in-depth scientific investigations on these fascinating yet somewhat elusive issues.

CULTURAL BELIEFS

Humans in general have an inherent need to make sense out of and explain their life experiences. This is especially true when they are experiencing suffering and illness. In the process of this quest for meaning, culturally shaped beliefs play a vital role in determining whether a particular explanation and associated treatment plan(s) will make sense to the patient and others in his or her social network or reference group. Numerous studies in medical anthropology have documented that "indigenous" systems of health beliefs and practices persist and may even flourish in all societies after their exposure to modern Western medicine (Kleinman 1980; Landy 1977). These beliefs and practices exert profound influences on patients' attitudes and behavior, and they often serve as the basis for the patients' perception of the causative factors associated with their illness and potential treatment options. These paradigms constructed by members of the nonmedically oriented public to explain their illness experiences have been termed "explanatory models." Although the power and importance of these lay explanatory models should be self-evident (Janz and Becker 1984; Kleinman 1988; Kleinman et al. 1978), they are often neglected in the clinical setting because of the power of socialization in the medical profession as well as deeply ingrained ethnocentrism and "medicocentrism." This incompatibility between lay and professional causal attributions, or explanatory models, often determines patients' satisfaction with treatment (Young and Garro 1982), medication compliance, and clinical outcome (Borkan et al. 1991; Weiss, in press).

For example, patients who are Hispanic or Asian often expect rapid relief from symptoms (Lin et al. 1991; Westermeyer 1989a), and they are generally cautious about potential detrimental side effects of Western medicine. These beliefs are possibly derived from their experiences with indigenous herbal drugs, which in general are less likely to induce side effects, as well as with modern analgesics and antibiotics, which typically provide quick relief of symptoms. These beliefs may also interfere with the patients' acceptance of modern-day psychopharmacologic treatment. Furthermore, the lengthy delay in noticeable improvement (inherent with most chronic psychiatric disorders) and the slow onset of action seen with many psychotropic medications (e.g., lithium, tricyclic antidepressants [TCAs], etc.) may lead patients to prematurely terminate their psychiatric care.

Concerns about the addictive and toxic effects of medication, which is often seen in patients who are Mexican (Martinez 1988) or Puerto Rican (Ramos-McKay et al. 1988), may lead to hesitancy about regularly taking medications for an indefinite time period (as is often the case with most psychotropics). On the other hand, because multiple herbal ingredients are usually prescribed by Asian practitioners of traditional medicine, Asian psychiatric patients often perceive the use of multiple drugs as more efficacious than single-drug therapy. Consequently, psychiatric patients in Japan are often treated in a fashion that would be regarded as polypharmacy in this country (Binder et al. 1987). The use of herbal or other organic ingredients as healing methods in other cultures warrants closer scrutiny by Western clinicians.

ISSUES INVOLVING SIMULTANEOUS USE OF TRADITIONAL AND/OR ALTERNATIVE HEALING METHODS

Despite the availability of Western-style medical services, traditional herbal medicines continue to be extensively used by Asians (Chan and Chang 1976; Kleinman 1980; Westermeyer 1989b), African-Americans (Vermeer and Farrell 1985), and Hispanics (Sankury 1983) living in the United States. Some of these herbal drugs have active pharmacologic properties that may interact with psychotropic drugs in different ways (Jones and Runikis 1987; Shader and Greenblatt 1988).

For example, the anticholinergic properties inherent in the Japanese herb *Swertia japonica* (Yamahara et al. 1991) and *kamikihi-to* (Egashira et al. 1991), or the Cuban folk medicine *Datura candida* (Carbajal et al. 1991) may cause atropine psychosis, particularly when ingested concomitantly with TCAs or low-potency neuroleptics. Because of its high concentration of caffeine, ingestion of the South American holly *Ilex guayusa* (Lewis et al. 1991) can complicate sedative hypnotic treatment. Concurrent use of the Nigerian root extract of *Schumanniophyton problematicum*, a popular treatment for psychosis among Nigerians (Amadi et al. 1991), with sedative hypnotics or neuroleptics may lead to potentiation of tranquilizing effects. In a recent study, several Chinese herbs, including *Fructus Schizandrae, Corydalis bungeane diels, Kopsia officinallis, Clausena lansium,* muscone, ginseng, and glycyrrhiza, have been found to have potent stimulating effects on the cytochrome P_{450} enzymes, and oleanolic acid contained in *Sertia mileensis* and *Ligustrum lucidium ait* substantially inhibits the activities of these enzymes (Liu 1991). Increased awareness and further clarification of these issues remain important as long as patients continue to rely on these traditional herbs as an adjunct to pharmacotherapy.

PATIENT COMPLIANCE

Successful treatment outcome is highly dependent on patient compliance with prescribed medications. It has been estimated, however, that at least 50% of patients do not adhere to physician instructions concerning their medication regimens (Sackett and Haynes 1976). The issues surrounding medication compliance are complicated, and compliance can affect measures of clinical outcome in many ways, including the following:

1. Patients may erroneously judge the efficaciousness of a treatment if noncompliance is followed by spontaneous cure;
2. Physicians may incorrectly judge the effectiveness and safety of the treatment if noncompliance is followed by improvement (Becker 1985); and
3. Interindividual variance with respect to compliance in clinical trials may cause investigators to reach incorrect conclusions about the superiority of one treatment over another.

Review articles by Sackett and Haynes (1976), Chen (1991), and Becker (1985) examined the compliance literature to identify factors that are most important in predicting noncompliance. Most of the earlier studies focused on patient attributes including sociodemographic variables, personality variables, and illness characteristics. These studies have resulted in conflicting findings. In contrast, studies focusing on the patient-clinician relationship, paying close attention to communication regarding drug actions and medication side effects, have yielded more useful results (Stimson 1974; Zola 1973). These studies demonstrated that patient's beliefs regarding the properties and effects contained in and exerted by medications are of central importance in determining compliance.

Clinicians treating cross-cultural patients must explore the beliefs held by their patients regarding illness causality and treatment expectations. Communication difficulties and divergence between patients and their treating professionals' explanatory models are at the heart of why ethnic minority patients are significantly more likely to drop out of psychiatric treatment (Acosta 1980; Sue and McKinney 1975). In a similar fashion, medication compliance with Western-oriented pharmacotherapy may be more problematic in cross-cultural settings. The results of a recent study in South Africa (Gillis et al. 1987) provide a dramatic example. In this study, 406 patients belonging to three ethnic groups (called "Whites," "Blacks," and "Colored") were followed for a 2-year period after discharge from a psychiatric hospital. They found that the noncompliance rate for oral phenothiazines was approximately two-thirds for Black patients, one-half for Colored patients, and one-quarter for White patients. Although the authors noted that the understanding of the treatment protocols by the relatives of the Black and Colored families was particularly poor, and entertained the possibility of culture and communication being significant factors contributing to the results, one must also consider the impact of structural barriers such as cost and availability of transportation, as well as discrimination. Perhaps for analogous reasons, African-Americans have been reported to be less compliant (D'Mello et al. 1989; Marcolin et al. 1991) and were consequently more likely to be placed on injectable antipsychotics (Price et al. 1985).

A study performed by Kinzie and colleagues (1987) serves to further illustrate problems with medication compliance in ethnic populations. The researchers found that 61% of their depressed refugee patients who were medicated showed no TCAs in their blood, and that another 24% revealed only very low TCA serum levels, even though all of them were treated with adequate TCA dosage. When questioned, these patients admitted not having been compliant for a variety of reasons. Education regarding the importance of long-term medication and the maintenance of appropriate blood levels resulted in significant improvement in compliance.

PLACEBO EFFECTS

Evaluating the efficacy of any treatment method, especially those involving the use of biological interventions, must include some measure of placebo effect. This phenomenon accounts for 30%–70% of the therapeutic responses observed with any treatment method. Although well recognized, the placebo effect has previously received minimal attention both in medical practice and in research (Kleinman 1988; White et al. 1985). Recently, reports have emerged that have provided useful information regarding the predictive value of factors such as diagnosis (Coryell and Noyes 1988; Loebel et al. 1986; Mavissakalian 1987, 1988; Mavissakalian et al. 1990; Spiker and Kupfer 1988), color, size, preparation, and method of drug administration (Buckalew and Coffield 1982; Buckalew and Ross 1981; Jacobs and Nordan 1979; Rabkin et al. 1990) on placebo responses.

By definition, placebo effects are mediated through "symbolic" rather than "instrumental" mechanisms and are thus expected to be largely influenced by culture (Lundh 1987; Moerman 1979). There is currently little specific information regarding how placebo responses might differ in various ethnic groups. In a multihospital collaborative study of phenothiazine treatment of schizophrenic psychoses, Goldberg and colleagues (1966) reported that African-American patients improved significantly more than their Caucasian counterparts. Escobar and Tuason (1980) conducted a cross-national study on the efficacy of trazodone and imipramine as compared with placebo in 40 Colombian and 32 American depressed patients. They found that the Colombian patients improved more than those in the United States not only with the antidepressants, but also when given placebo. Although the number of the studies precludes any firm conclusions, available data appear to suggest that non-Caucasians may be somewhat more responsive to placebo treatment. In another study, Buckalew and Coffield (1982) reported ethnic differences in response to the color and preparation of placebo. Such differences were most striking when comparing white and black capsules. White capsules were seen as analgesics by Caucasian subjects but as stimulants by African-American subjects; in contrast, black capsules were seen as stimulants by Caucasians and as analgesics by African-Americans. Although the symbolic meaning of this finding was not explored in this study, the culture- and ethnic-specific nature concerning drug effects appears self-evident.

Although empirical data are not available, clinical lore has long suggested that Asians often express "excessive" concerns about the side effects of psychotropics (Lin and Shen 1991). This concern may lead to placebo side effects and to subsequent discontinuation or lowering of the drug dosage. To what extent this is true remains to be investigated. In a detailed longitudinal study of side effects reported by 57 Hong Kong Chinese psychiatric patients receiving lithium, Lee (in press) identified cultural influences in the concern and reporting of untoward symptoms attributed to lithium by these patients. In contrast to Western patients, Chinese patients rarely complained of "missing of highs," "loss of creativity," weight gain, or a metallic taste in their mouths. Although polydipsia and polyuria were present in the majority of these patients, these side effects were positively, not negatively, interpreted. Complaints such as lethargy, poor memory, and drowsiness appeared to be related to the fear the subjects had of not being able to work, and actually occurred at a similar frequency as age- and sex-matched control subjects. This study clearly demonstrated the importance of cultural beliefs in patients' interpretation and reporting of side effects.

PERSONALITY STYLES AND DRUG RESPONSE

In the early days of the "psychotropic era" (during the 1960s and early 1970s), many clinical reports (Janke 1983; Murphy 1969; Slater and Kastenbaum 1966) suggested that personality traits may significantly influence psychotropic responses in patients as well as control subjects (Janke 1983). These studies, typically involving the use of sedating agents such as low-potency neuroleptics, barbiturates, and benzodiazepines, suggested that personality traits may significantly influence subjects' response to these medications. Those who responded in an "orthodox" manner (i.e., sedation) tended to be passive and intellectually oriented, whereas those who experienced "paradoxical reactions" to these drugs were typically "action-oriented" and athletically inclined. Their responses were often characterized by a paradoxical increase in agitation, tension, and anxiety. Although most of these studies were flawed in their study designs, they did point out an important area of research that merits closer scrutiny.

Although phenomenal progress has occurred in the biological areas of psychopharmacological research, these "softer" issues have been brushed aside and largely forgotten. Despite this neglect, reports associating personality with psychotropic responses have continued to sporadically appear in the literature (Shawcross and Tyrer 1985). Some of these reports have demonstrated findings suggesting that personality traits may substantially influence the pharmacodynamics of psychotropics (Janke 1983; Kawazu et al. 1980; Parrott and Kentridge 1982). Recent reports further substantiate a significant correlation between personality traits and the pharmacogenetic (Bertilsson et al. 1989) and pharmacokinetic (Nakano et al. 1980) characteristics of study subjects.

Through the process of childrearing and socialization, culture is commonly regarded as an important factor in shaping the personality structure of individuals. It is conceivable that, in addition to the pharmacokinetic and pharmacodynamic factors discussed in previous chapters, culturally related differences in "normative" personality traits could represent another mechanism that may have some importance in determining ethnic differences in drug responses. Along this line of reasoning, earlier researchers have speculated about some of the observed differences in psychotropic response between Westerners and non-Westerners. One hypothesis (Murphy 1969, 1972) suggested that Westerners might be less responsive to sedating drugs because they tend to be more "action-oriented," and thus require higher doses of these medications to achieve desired effect. It is clear that without empirical data to support or refute these hypotheses, these important issues will remain speculative and unclarified at best (Lin et al. 1990).

SOCIAL SUPPORT SYSTEMS

The structure and function of social networks are thought to influence the prognosis and outcome of treatment of people who are mentally ill. Research has demonstrated that a person who loses his or her social support through death of a spouse, divorce, or isolation from relocation is much more likely to become mentally ill (Lidwig and Collete 1970; Mishler and Scotch 1963; Myers et al. 1972), and less likely to be compliant with prescribed medication (Nelson et al. 1980). In addition, recent studies have further suggested that alterations in the level of stress and the availability of social support may also change the therapeutic dosages and therapeutic concentration ranges of different psychotropics. For example, Lieberman and Strauss (1984) recently demonstrated that bipolar patients experienced relapses despite adequate lithium treatment while they were subjected to intense interpersonal conflicts. These episodes were brought under control only when the patients' lithium dosages and concentrations were raised beyond the ranges previously found adequate.

Three areas of ethnic differences in the nature of social support are of particular importance.

Extent of Involvement and Support

Ethnicity definitely exerts strong influences on the way family members interact with patients (Jenkins and Karno 1992; Kinzie and Bolton 1973; Kirmayer and Robbins 1991; Lin 1987; McGoldrick et al. 1982). For example, in a study comparing the response of 26 Asian and 26 Caucasian schizophrenic patients to haloperidol treatment, Lin and colleagues (1991) found that 19 Asians versus 4 Caucasians were accompanied by family members at the time of initial assessment. During the 3-month treatment course, 25 Asians versus 12 Caucasians had some type of family involvement in their treatment. This is supported by a study by Nunez (1976), who found that among Hispanic and Caucasian inpatients, Hispanics had a greater frequency of interaction with relatives and became more demoralized when such interaction did not take place. These differences in family involvement may have relevance in treatment outcome. For example, two large-scale, multinational follow-up studies of the outcome of schizophrenia sponsored by the World Health Organization (WHO; Jablensky et al. 1992; Lin and Kleinman 1988; WHO 1979) consistently revealed that non-Western patients had more social support and also had significantly better clinical outcome as compared to their Western counterparts.

Structure of the Social Network

Two types of support networks have been described in the literature: "open" and "closed." Americans who are Caucasian typically engage in "open" support networks, consisting of a large number of people with weak connections to each other (i.e., few know or relate to each other in the network). "Closed" support networks consist of family members, kin, and intimate friends who have all known each other over a long period of time; this type of network has been reported to be typical of Hispanics and Asians (Comas-Diaz and Griffith 1988; Martinez 1978). As discussed previously, the "closed" social networks often are more able to provide patients with effective support conducive to emotional well-being as well as recovery from severe mental illness. Although such social networks have a positive impact on the care of mentally ill patients, they may also have some negative influence, including delay in help-seeking outside of the patients' local community as well as problems with compliance.

Quality of Support

In addition to the structure of the network and the intensity of involvement of other people, the type and quality of the interaction between network members may also vary cross-culturally. For example, limited research data have suggested that Caucasian American families are more likely to be rated as having high expressed emotion (EE) compared to their British counterparts, and Hispanic families tend to have significantly lower EE ratings as compared to Caucasian Americans and Caucasian Britons (Jenkins and Karno 1992; Keefe et al. 1978). Several well-designed studies examining the effect of EE have found that patients with high-EE family members (characterized by frequent criticism, hostility, and emotional overinvolvement) were significantly more likely to relapse on standard neuroleptic doses (Anderson et al. 1986; Falloon et al. 1984) and to be subsequently treated with higher doses of the same medication (Falloon and Liberman 1983; Hogarty et al. 1988). It is possible that such cultural differences in family atmosphere may have important influences on drug responsiveness across cultures.

DIAGNOSTIC ISSUES

Psychiatric diagnosis and case formulation is a difficult and complicated process when evaluating cross-cultural patients (Lin and Shen 1991). Identifying target symptoms that warrant pharmacological treatment is the critical first step in the selection of psychotropic medications. An inappropriate therapeutic regimen prescribed as a result of diagnostic error is more than likely to result in the development of untoward side effects and/or worsening of the patient's illness. The emergence of bothersome side effects can therefore adversely influence patient satisfaction and future compliance. Considering the importance of diagnosis for appropriate pharmacotherapy, mental health practitioners should understand the barriers to accurate diagnostic assessment of cross-cultural patients. The most important impediments encountered in the evaluation of minority patients previously identified by several authors include differences with respect to language, communication style, and cultural beliefs (Kleinman 1988; Thompson and Thompson 1990; Tseng and McDermott 1981; Westermeyer 1985, 1989b).

Language Issues

Language plays a critical role in the evaluation of ethnic minorities (Russell 1988). Flaskerud and Hu (1992) reported that 60% of Asians and 50% of Hispanics studied in the Los Angeles mental health system did not speak English. In the presence of a significant language barrier, a successful psychiatric interview requires the services of either a bilingual mental health practitioner or a translator. If neither is available and/or a clinical exigency exists, the evaluator may be forced to proceed despite these limitations.

Practitioners who are not bilingual must be aware of problems that may arise when evaluating a patient who speaks little English. Potential mental status irregularities may be observed in such a patient that may be more a product of difficulties involved in thinking in one language and talking in another rather than evidence of thought-processing problems (Marcos 1979). For example, as the patient hesitates and searches for a word, he or she may appear to be experiencing thought blocking, thought derailment, or looseness of associations. Similarly, a patient who is unable to easily express thoughts or emotions secondary to a limited vocabulary may appear to have paucity of thought or blunted affect.

Although the use of medically trained interpreters is encouraged, when they are unavailable, a member of the patient's family or a bilingual friend is often called upon to act as translator. Such practices may produce other pitfalls in diagnostic assessment. First, family members may be invested in a particular evaluation outcome and may alter the patient's comments in translation. Minimizing or exaggerating the patient's verbalized content and symptomatology may represent efforts to avoid the stigma of a psychiatric label or to ensure hospitalization, respectively. Second, patients may feel uncomfortable discussing certain symptoms or issues (e.g., child, spouse, or elder abuse) with the evaluator in the presence of a family member acting as translator. Finally, when family members and significant others act as interpreters, they tend to make errors of omission, addition, condensation, substitution, and role exchange, all of which can lead to inaccuracies in the diagnosis (Faust and Drickery 1986; Marcos 1979; Vasquez and Javier 1991).

Diagnostic accuracy is clearly increased when bilingual mental health practitioners perform evaluations of monolingual or bilingual cross-cultural patients. However, a cautionary note must be extended in the case of bilingual clients. The nature and severity of the psychopathology may differ between interviews conducted in the patient's primary language and those in a second language (Marcos 1979).

Communication Style

Significant diversity exists between and among cultures in styles of communication (Arce 1982; Fitzpatrick and Gould 1970; Hall 1976) that can affect both the diagnosis as well as the doctor-patient relationship. The direct communication style of Caucasian Americans is in direct contrast to the more reserved and less expressive style often encountered with Hispanic and Asian patients (Falicov 1982; Lin and Shen 1991). Direct questioning, informal use of language, and insistence on full disclosure may lead to increased suspiciousness and difficulty in establishing good rapport between doctor and patient.

Nonverbal communication is a highly developed form of social interaction in some ethnic minority groups. For example, a certain smile or nervous laugh may be used to hide displeasure, anger, or sorrow among Japanese (Morsbach 1973). Among Southeast Asian refugees and rural African-Americans, extensive direct eye contact is considered rude and disrespectful. Touching the head of a Southeast Asian refugee should also be avoided if possible, because it is considered the sacred resting place of the soul. The use of a common American hand gesture (palm up with fingers motioning toward the speaker's body) to usher a refugee patient into a room can be interpreted as insulting and disrespectful because such a gesture may be used in the patient's native country to beckon to young children and animals.

Cultural Issues

Culture affects not only how the patient experiences illness (Gerson 1976) but also which symptoms he or she feels warrant medical attention (Mechanic 1975). For example, though a significant number of Asian, African, and Hispanic depressive patients focus on somatic complaints (Mezzich and Raab 1980), Caucasian Americans complain more often of the suicidal manifestations associated with depressive illness (Mezzich and Raab 1980).

Culturally naive evaluators may diagnose delusional thinking in a patient when ideas or beliefs that are culturally shaped are expressed as etiological explanations for symptomatology. Among blacks, Hispanics, and American Indians, the concepts of spiritual possession, sorcery, and witchcraft are often culturally used to explain mental illness (Alonso and Jeffrey 1988; Beiser 1985; Campinha-Bacote 1992; Edgerton 1966; Mail et al. 1989). Lastly, cultural differences between patient and therapist can further confuse a nonminority therapist by introducing information that is out of the realms of his or her experience. A black or Hispanic patient who lives in a neighborhood where gang violence is prevalent reporting a fear of being shot by strangers is more than likely describing reality-based fear rather than paranoia. In a similar fashion, the Southeast Asian, Mexican, or Central American refugee who talks of witnessing or being the victim of horrible atrocities may also be inappropriately labeled with a major Axis I psychopathological disorder (Cervantes et al. 1989; Hall 1988; Lin and Shen 1991).

CONCLUSIONS AND SUGGESTIONS FOR FUTURE RESEARCH

Although systematic research employing careful study design has not been conducted to evaluate these important issues, clinical reports and limited empirical data indicate that sociocultural forces shape the nature of "nonbiological" factors that appear to influence how patients respond to psychotropics. To go beyond these broad generalizations, however, more sophisticated and innovative research designs will be needed. Progress in these areas has been impeded by the complexity and subjectivity involved in the interaction of culture and psychopharmacology. Several recent developments may make these obstacles less formidable. Cross-cultural validity of psychiatric diagnosis, although still far from perfect, has improved substantially in recent years and will help to ensure the comparability of patients enrolled in such studies. Also, progress in pharmacokinetics and pharmacodynamics makes it relatively easier to separate "nonbiological" from biological effects of psychotropics and will serve to substantially reduce the ambiguity that confronted researchers in the past. Such advances in methodology should enable researchers to explore innovative approaches to further our understanding on these important issues. Possible study designs include the following:

1. Compliance and its social and clinical correlates could be more accurately assessed in longitudinal follow-up studies of patients with different ethnic backgrounds but with similar diagnosis and treatment.
2. Biological measurements (e.g., drug serum concentrations) could be useful in the identification of noncompliance and placebo response.
3. Phase III (placebo-controlled, double-blind testing) of the efficacy studies of drugs being developed for marketing could be designed to include multiple ethnic comparison groups.
4. The treatment response data from these Phase III efficacy studies could then be used for ethnic comparison of issues involving the "nonbiological" variables discussed in this chapter.

The need for future research notwithstanding, the literature as reviewed does consistently suggest several practical guidelines that should be useful for clinicians treating cross-cultural patients.

1. Information regarding patients' beliefs about their illnesses and what constitutes effective treatment (their explanatory models) should be elicited on a routine basis. Symptoms that have significant meaning to the patients should not be neglected.
2. Patients' beliefs in traditional and/or alternative medical practices, such as the use of herbs, should also be routinely elicited. If herb-drug interaction is suspected, the active ingredients of these herbs should be investigated by consulting cultural experts and/or specialists in pharmacognosy.
3. Treatment plans should be explained in culturally meaningful ways. This should greatly facilitate patient-clinician communication and raise the level of mutual trust and respect, thus enhancing the drug's efficacy by facilitating compliance as well as the occurrence of the placebo effects.
4. Compliance issues should be discussed with patients and their family members in a supportive and open manner. These discussions should be aimed at educating both patient and family members about psychotropic medication drug actions and side effects. Regular monitoring of serum or plasma drug concentrations may be performed as an adjunct to ensure level of compliance.
5. In most cases, key family members should be included in discussions regarding diagnoses and treatment planning.

REFERENCES

Acosta FX: Self-described reasons for premature termination of psychotherapy by Mexican American, Black American, and Anglo-American patients. Psychol Rep 47:435–443, 1980

Alonso L, Jeffrey WD: Mental illness complicated by the Santeria belief in spirit possession. Hosp Community Psychiatry 39:1188–1191, 1988

Amadi E, Offiah NV, Akah PA: Neuropyschopharmacologic properties of a Schumanniophyton problematicum root extract. J Ethnopharmacol 33:73–77, 1991

Anderson CM, Reiss DJ, Hogarty GE (eds): Schizophrenia and the Family: A Practitioner's Guide to Psychoeducation and Management. New York, Guilford, 1986

Arce AA: Psychiatric training issues: the Puerto Rican perspective. Am J Psychiatry 129:461–465, 1982
Becker MH: Patient adherence to prescribed therapies. Med Care 23:539–555, 1985
Becker M, Maiman LA: Strategies for enhancing patient compliance. J Community Health 6:113–135, 1980
Beiser M: The grieving witch: a framework for applying principles of cultural psychiatry to clinical practice. Can J Psychiatry 30:130–141, 1985
Bertilsson L, Alm C, De Las Carreras C, et al: Debrisoquine hydroxylation polymorphism and personality. Lancet 1:555, 1989
Binder RL, Kazamatsuri H, Nishimura T, et al: Tardive dyskinesia and neuroleptic-induced parkinsonism in Japan. Am J Psychiatry 144:1494–1496, 1987
Borkan JM, Quirk M, Sullivan M: Finding meaning after the fall: injury narratives from elderly hip fracture patients. Soc Sci Med 33(8):947–957, 1991
Buckalew LW, Coffield KE: Drug expectations associated with perceptual characteristics: ethnic factors. Percept Mot Skills 55:915–918, 1982
Buckalew LW, Ross S: Relationship of perceptual characteristics to efficacy of placebos. Psychol Rep 49:955–961, 1981
Campinha-Bacote J: Voodoo illness. Perspect Psychiatr Care 28:11–17, 1992
Carbajal D, Casaco A, Arruzazabala L, et al: Pharmacological screening of plant decoctions commonly used in Cuban folk medicine. J Ethnopharmacol 33:21–24, 1991
Cervantes RC, Salgado de Snyder VN, Padilla AM: Posttraumatic stress in immigrants from Central America and Mexico. Hosp Community Psychiatry 40:615–619, 1989
Chan CW, Chang JK: The role of Chinese medicine in New York City's Chinatown. Am J Chinese Med 4:31–45, 129–146, 1976
Chen A: Noncompliance in community psychiatry: a review of clinical interventions. Hosp Community Psychiatry 42:282–287, 1991
Comas-Diaz L, Griffith EEH (eds): Clinical Guidelines in Cross-Cultural Mental Health. New York, Wiley, 1988
Coryell W, Noyes R: Placebo response in panic disorder. Am J Psychiatry 145:1138, 1988
D'Mello DA, McNeil JA, Harris W: Multiethnic variance in psychiatric diagnosis and neuroleptic dosage. Paper presented at the annual meeting of the American Psychiatric Association, San Francisco, CA, May 6–11, 1989

Edgerton RB: Conceptions of psychosis in four East African societies. American Anthropologist 68:409–423, 1966
Egashira T, Sudo S, Murayama F, et al: Effects of kamikihi-to, a Chinese traditional medicine, on various cholinergic biochemical markers in the brain of aged rats. Folia Pharmacologica Japonica 98:273–281, 1991
Escobar JI, Tuason VB: Antidepressant agents: a cross cultural study. Psychopharmacol Bull 16:49–52, 1980
Falicov CJ: Mexican families, in Ethnicity and Family Therapy. Edited by McGoldrick M, Pearce JK, Giordano J. New York, Guilford, 1982, pp 134–163
Falloon IRH, Liberman RP: Interactions between drug and psychosocial therapy in schizophrenia. Schizophr Bull 9:543–554, 1983
Falloon IRH, Boyd JL, McGill CW (eds): Family Care of Schizophrenia: A Problem-Solving Approach to the Treatment of Mental Illness. New York, Guilford, 1984
Faust S, Drickery R: Working with interpreters. J Fam Pract 22:131–138, 1986
Fitzpatrick JP, Gould RE: Mental illness among Puerto Ricans in New York: cultural or intercultural misunderstanding? Am J Orthopsychiatry 40:238–239, 1970
Flaskerud JH, Hu L: Racial/ethnic identity and amount and type of psychiatric treatment. Am J Psychiatry 149:379–384, 1992
Gerson EM: The social character of illness: deviance or politics? Soc Sci Med 10:219–224, 1976
Gillis LS, Trollip D, Jakoet A, et al: Non-compliance with psychotropic medication. S Afr Med J 72:602–606, 1987
Goldberg SC, Schooler NR, Davidson EM, et al: Sex and race differences in response to drug treatment among schizophrenics. Psychopharmacologia (Berlin) 9:31–47, 1966
Hall ET: Beyond Culture. Garden City, NY, Encore/Doubleday, 1976
Hall LK Sr: Providing culturally relevant mental health services for Central American immigrants. Hosp Community Psychiatry 39:1139, 1988
Hogarty GE, McEvoy JP, Munetz M, et al: Dose of fluphenazine, familial expressed emotion, and outcome in schizophrenia. Arch Gen Psychiatry 45:797–805, 1988
Jablensky A, Sartorius N, Ernberg G, et al: Schizophrenia: manifestations, incidence and course in different cultures: a World Health Organization ten-country study. Psychol Med Monogr Suppl 20:1–97, 1992
Jacobs KW, Nordan FM: Classification of placebo drugs: effect of color. Percept Mot Skills 49:367–372, 1979

Janke W: Response variability to psychotropic drugs: overview of the main approaches to differential pharmacopsychology, in Response Variability to Psychotropic Drugs. Edited by Janke W. New York, Pergamon, 1983, pp 217–260

Janz NK, Becker MH: The health belief model a decade later. Health Educ Q 11:1–47, 1984

Jenkins JH, Karno M: The meaning of expressed emotion: theoretical issues raised by cross-cultural research. Am J Psychiatry 149:9–21, 1992

Jones BD, Runikis AM: Interaction of ginseng with phenelzine. J Clin Psychopharmacol 201–202, 1987

Kawazu Y, Nakano S, Ogawa N: Personality trait and antianxiety drug effects on psychomotor performance. Neuropsychopharmacol 4:285–292, 1980

Keefe SE, Padilla AM, Carlos ML: Emotional support systems in two cultures: a comparison of Mexican-Americans and Anglo Americans. Los Angeles, CA, University of California, Spanish Speaking Mental Health Center, 1978

Kinzie JD, Bolton JM: Psychiatry with the Aborigines of West Malaysia. Am J Psychiatry 130:769–773, 1973

Kinzie JD, Leung P, Boehnlein J, et al: Tricyclic antidepressant plasma levels in Indochinese refugees: clinical implication. J Nerv Ment Dis 175:480–485, 1987

Kirmayer LJ, Robbins JM: Current Concepts of Somatization: Research and Clinical Perspectives (Progress in Psychiatry #31). Washington, DC, American Psychiatric Press, 1991

Kleinman A: Patients and Healers in the Context of Culture. Berkeley, CA, University of California Press, 1980

Kleinman A: Rethinking Psychiatry. New York, Free Press, 1988

Kleinman A, Eisenberg L, Good B: Culture, illness, and cure. Ann Intern Med 88:251–258, 1978

Landy D (ed): Culture, Disease, and Healing: Studies in Medical Anthropology. New York, Macmillan, 1977

Lee S: Side effects of lithium therapy in Hong Kong Chinese: an ethnopsychiatric perspective. Cult Psychiatry Med (in press)

Lewis WH, Kennelly EJ, Bass GN, et al: Ritualistic use of the holly Ilex guayusa by Amazonian Jivaro Indians. J Ethnopharmacol 33:25–30, 1991

Lidwig EG, Collete J: Dependency, social isolation and mental health in a disabled population. Social Psychiatry 5:92–95, 1970

Lieberman PB, Strauss JS: The recurrence of mania: environmental factors and medical treatment. Am J Psychiatry 141:77–80, 1984

Lin KM: Experiences on inpatient wards: Taiwan vs Los Angeles. American Journal of Social Psychiatry 7:220–225, 1987

Lin KM, Kleinman AM: Psychopathology and clinical course of schizophrenia: a cross-cultural perspective. Schizophr Bull 14:555–567, 1988

Lin KM, Shen WW: Pharmacotherapy for Southeast Asian psychiatric patients. J Nerv Ment Dis 179:346–350, 1991

Lin KM, Poland RE, Chien CP: Ethnicity and psychopharmacology: recent findings and future research directions, in Family, Culture and Psychobiology. Edited by Sorel E. New York, Legas, 1990, pp 111–131

Lin KM, Miller MM, Nuccio I, et al: Ethnicity and family involvement in the treatment of schizophrenic patients. J Nerv Ment Dis 179:626–628, 1991

Liu GT: Effects of some compounds isolated from Chinese medicinal herbs on hepatic microsomal cytochrome P-450 and their potential biological consequences. Drug Metab Rev 23:439–465, 1991

Loebel AD, Hyde TS, Dunner DL: Early placebo response in anxious and depressed patients. J Clin Psychiatry 47:230–233, 1986

Lundh L-G: Placebo, belief, and health: a cognitive-emotional model. Scand J Psychol 28:128–143, 1987

Mail PD, McKay RB, Katz M: Expanding practice horizons: learning from American Indian patients. Patient Education and Counseling 13:91–102, 1989

Marcolin MA, Stiers W, Chung YS: Racial differences in schizophrenia when controlling for economic status (Continuing Medical Education Syllabus and Scientific Proceedings, pp 80–81). Paper presented at the annual meeting of the American Psychiatric Association, New Orleans, LA, May 11–16, 1991

Marcos LR: Effects of interpreters on the evaluation of psychopathology in non-English-speaking patients. Am J Psychiatry 136:171–174, 1979

Martinez C: Mexican-Americans, in Clinical Guidelines in Cross-Cultural Mental Health. Edited by Comas-Diaz L, Griffith EEH. New York, Wiley, 1988, pp 182–183

Martinez RA (ed): Hispanic Culture and Health Care: Fact, Fiction, and Folklore. St. Louis, MO, CV Mosby, 1978

Mavissakalian M: The placebo effect in agoraphobia. J Nerv Ment Dis 175:95–99, 1987

Mavissakalian M: The placebo effect in agoraphobia—II. J Nerv Ment Dis 176:446–448, 1988

Mavissakalian MR, Jones B, Olson S: Absence of placebo response in obsessive-compulsive disorder. J Nerv Ment Dis 178:268–270, 1990

McGoldrick M, Pearce JK, Giordano J (eds): Ethnicity and Family Therapy. New York, Guilford, 1982

Mechanic D: Sociocultural and social-psychological factors affecting personal responses to psychological disorder. J Health Soc Behav 16:393–404, 1975

Mezzich JE, Raab ES: Depressive symptomatology across the Americas. Arch Gen Psychiatry 37:818–823, 1980

Mishler EG, Scotch NA: Sociocultural factors in the epidemiology of schizophrenia: a review. Psychiatry 26:315–351, 1963

Moerman DE: Anthropology of symbolic healing. Currents in Anthropology 20:59–80, 1979

Morsbach H: Aspects of nonverbal communication in Japan. J Nerv Ment Dis 157:262–277, 1973

Murphy HBM: Ethnic variations in drug responses. Transcultural Psychiatric Research Review 6:6–23, 1969

Murphy HBM: Psychopharmacologie et variations ethnoculturelles. Confrontation Psychiatrique 9:163–185, 1972

Myers JK, Jacob JL, Pepper MD, et al: Life events and mental status: a longitudinal study. J Health Soc Behav 13:398–406, 1972

Nakano S, Ogawa N, Kawazu Y: Influence of neuroticism on oral absorption of diazepam. Clin Pharmacol Ther 27:370–374, 1980

Nelson E, Stason W, Neutra R, et al: Identification of noncompliant hypertensive patients. Prev Med 9:504–517, 1980

Nunez F: Variations in fulfillment of expectations of social interaction and morale among aging Mexican-Americans and Anglos. Master's Thesis, University of Southern California, 1976

Parrott AC, Kentridge R: Personal constructs of anxiety under the 1,5-benzodiazepine derivative clobazam related to trait-anxiety levels of the personality. Psychopharmacology (Berlin) 78:353–357, 1982

Price N, Glazer W, Morgenstern H: Demographic predictors of the use of injectable versus oral antipsychotic medications in outpatients. Am J Psychiatry 142:1491–1492, 1985

Rabkin JG, McGrath PJ, Quitkin FM, et al: Effects of pill-giving on maintenance of placebo response in patients with chronic mild depression. Am J Psychiatry 147:1622–1626, 1990

Ramos-McKay JM, Comas-Diaz L, Rivera LA: Puerto Ricans, in Clinical Guidelines in Cross-Cultural Mental Health. Edited by Comas-Diaz L, Griffith EEH. New York, Wiley, 1988, pp 204–232

Russell DM: Language and psychotherapy: the influence of nonstandard English in clinical practice, in Clinical Guidelines in Cross-Cultural Mental Health. Edited by Comas-Diaz L, Griffith EEH. New York, Wiley, 1988, pp 33–68

Sackett DL, Haynes RB (eds): Compliance With Therapeutic Regimens. Baltimore, MD, Johns Hopkins University Press, 1976

Sankury T: Lead poisoning from Mexican folk remedies—California (letter). JAMA 250:3149, 1983

Shader RI, Greenblatt DJ: Bees, ginseng and MAOI's revisited. J Clin Psychopharmacol 8:325, 1988

Shawcross CR, Tyrer P: Influence of personality on response to monoamine oxidase inhibitors and tricyclic antidepressants. J Psychiatr Res 19:557–562, 1985

Slater PE, Kastenbaum R: Paradoxical reactions to drugs: some personality and ethnic correlates. J Am Geriatr Soc 14:1016–1034, 1966

Spiker DG, Kupfer DJ: Placebo response rates in psychotic and nonpsychotic depression. J Affect Disord 14:21–23, 1988

Stimson GV: Obeying doctor's orders: a view from the other side. Soc Sci Med 8:97–104, 1974

Sue S, McKinney H: Asian-Americans in the community mental health care system. Am J Orthopsychiatry 45:11–118, 1975

Thompson WL, Thompson TL II: Taking care of culturally different and non-English speaking patients. Int J Psychiatry Med 20:235–245, 1990

Tseng WS, McDermott JF Jr: Culture, Mind and Therapy: An Introduction to Cultural Psychiatry. New York, Brunner/Mazel, 1981

Vasquez C, Javier RA: The problem with interpreters: communicating with Spanish-speaking patients. Hosp Community Psychiatry 42:163–165, 1991

Vermeer DE, Farrell RE: Nigerian geophagical clay: a traditional antidiarrheal pharmaceutical. Science 227:634–636, 1985

Weiss M: The explanatory model interview catalogue (EMIC): contribution to cross-cultural research methods from a study of leprosy and mental health. Br J Psychiatry (in press)

Westermeyer J: Psychiatric diagnosis across cultural boundaries. Am J Psychiatry 142:7, 1985

Westermeyer J: Psychiatric Care of Migrants: A Clinical Guide. Washington, DC, American Psychiatric Press, 1989a

Westermeyer J: Mental Health for Refugees and Other Migrants. Springfield, IL, Charles C Thomas, 1989b

White L, Tursky B, Schwartz GE (eds): Placebo—Theory, Research and Mechanisms. New York, Guilford, 1985

World Health Organization: Schizophrenia: An International Follow-up Study. Chichester, England, Wiley, 1979

Yamahara J, Kobayashi M, Matsuda H, et al: Anticholinergic action of Swertia Japonica and an active constituent. J Ethnopharmacol 33:31–35, 1991

Young J, Garro LY: Variation in the choice of treatment in two Mexican communities. Soc Sci Med 16:1463–1466, 1982

Zola IK: Pathways to the doctor—from person to patient. Soc Sci Med 7:677–684, 1973

Section II

Ethnicity and Psychopharmacology

Chapter 4

Ethnicity and the Pharmacology of Tricyclic Antidepressants

Barbara Silver, M.D., Russell E. Poland, Ph.D., and Keh-Ming Lin, M.D., M.P.H.

Since the development and availability of tricyclic antidepressants (TCAs) in the 1950s, these agents have become the cornerstone of biological therapy for unipolar depressive illness. In addition, the TCAs have been widely used in the treatment of bipolar disorder, anxiety disorders such as panic disorder and obsessive-compulsive disorder, childhood disorders such as attention-deficit hyperactivity disorder and enuresis, eating disorders, and chronic pain syndromes. Clinical observations have suggested that people of different ethnic backgrounds may respond differently to TCAs. As these agents are prescribed throughout the world and as most metropolitan areas have become increasingly multiethnic, the optimal use of TCAs demands a further understanding of the nature of any ethnic differences in the pharmacology of TCAs, as well as an understanding of the origins of these dissimilarities. Certain questions must then be answered: Do people of various ethnicities respond differently to the same dose of TCAs, both with respect to clinical efficacy and side effects? If so, are these variations determined by kinetic factors (such as protein binding, metabolism, and excretion) that determine plasma TCA concentrations, or are they determined by dynamic factors, such as drug-receptor interactions?

In this chapter, we examine the potential etiologies of ethnic

Supported in part by Research Center on the Psychobiology of Ethnicity MH47193 (Drs. Lin and Poland) and National Institute of Mental Health Research Scientist Development Award MH00534 (Dr. Poland).

differences in the pharmacology of TCAs, including a discussion of pharmacokinetic variables such as protein binding and drug metabolism, as well as pharmacodynamic factors such as drug-receptor interactions. A particular focus is on metabolic factors influencing steady-state concentrations of TCAs, because it is these concentrations, and not the dosages administered, that are more important determinants of clinical efficacy and side effects (Asberg et al. 1970, 1971; Sjoqvist et al. 1971). We then review the literature on TCAs and ethnicity (including clinical impressions, single-dose kinetic studies in control subjects, and clinical studies in patients) and discuss directions for future research.

PHARMACOKINETICS OF TCAs

Protein Binding of TCAs

TCAs are extensively protein-bound, and—as with many other medications—it is the unbound fraction that is biologically active, contributing to both clinical efficacy and side effects. Ethnic variations in protein binding have been found for nonpsychiatric medications, including the antihistamine diphenhydramine (Spector et al. 1980) and the antihypertensive propranolol (Zhou et al. 1989).

Specifically regarding TCAs, Borga and colleagues (1969) found that at least 90% of TCAs are protein-bound, with the tertiary amines amitriptyline (AT) and imipramine (IMI) being bound in higher percentages than their corresponding metabolites nortriptyline (NT) and desipramine (DMI). TCA protein binding remains relatively constant over a wide range of plasma TCA concentrations, with little interindividual difference in protein binding (Borga et al. 1969). In a study of twins, Alexanderson and Borga (1972) found a twofold variation in the binding ratio of NT to plasma proteins, with variance within pairs being greater for dizygotic than monozygotic twins. Even within monozygotic twins, differences were significant, indicating both genetic and environmental influences. However, this twofold variation is minor when compared with differences in TCA steady-state concentrations that exist, as described in the next section. Regarding ethnic differences, Rudorfer and colleagues (1984) did not find differences in protein binding of DMI between Caucasian and Chinese volunteer subjects in the United States, possibly due to similarities in the environments of the two groups.

Metabolism of TCAs

After oral administration, TCAs undergo extensive first-pass metabolism to both active and inactive metabolites, markedly reducing systemic availability. The TCAs have a large volume of distribution (V_d), as they are strongly bound to plasma proteins and to tissues. Metabolism that occurs prior to renal elimination includes demethylation and hydroxylation (under the control of hepatic cytochrome P_{450} enzymes) followed by glucuronide conjugation to form water-soluble compounds. (See Figure 4–1 for a schematic of TCA metabolism). Specifically, the tertiary amines AT and IMI are N-demethylated to form their respective secondary amines NT and DMI; AT and NT are hydroxylated preferentially at the 10 position, whereas IMI and DMI are hydroxylated preferentially at the 2 position. Both genetic and environmental variables may influence TCA metabolism and thus will be discussed in detail.

Environmental variables have been found to influence drug metabolism, including but not limited to concomitant drug therapy, diet, smoking, caffeine intake, and exposure to alcohol. Specifically regarding TCAs, medications that lower TCA concentrations through hepatic enzyme induction include contraceptive hormones, other steroids, and barbiturates (Balderassini 1985; Hammer and Sjoqvist 1967). Drugs that increase TCA concentrations include phenothiazines, stimulants, certain antibiotics (Balderassini 1985), and the antidepressant fluoxetine (Downs and Dahmer 1990; Downs et al. 1989; Preskorn et al. 1990; Rosenstein et al. 1991; von Ammon Cavanaugh 1990). The interaction of fluoxetine with TCAs has been linked to inhibition of TCA hydroxylation by fluoxetine and its major metabolite, norfluoxetine (Brosen and Skjelbo 1991). Such drug interactions must not be ignored in psychiatric patients, many of whom are treated with multiple medications. More importantly, prescribing practices vary throughout the world, compounding the possibility for environmental influences on TCA metabolism.

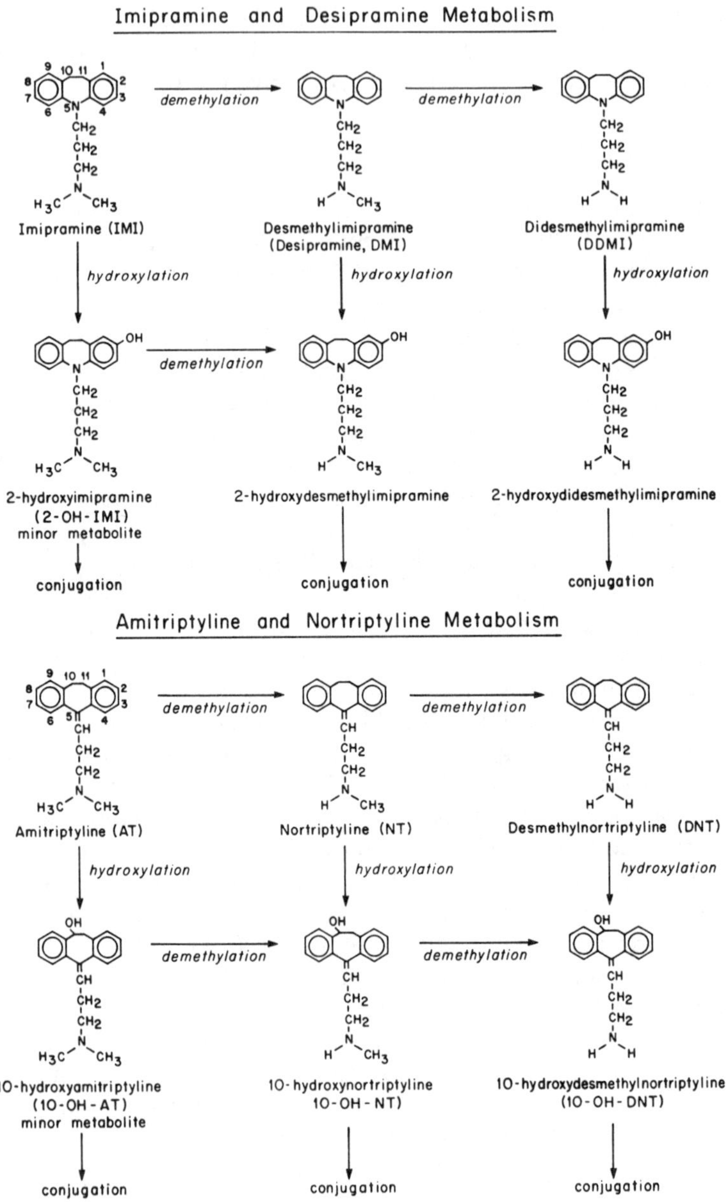

Figure 4–1. Major pathways of tricyclic antidepressant metabolism.

Steady-state TCA plasma concentrations have been shown to vary widely among individuals; however, in given individuals such concentrations remain constant over time (Potter et al. 1981; Sjoqvist et al. 1971). Significantly, drug concentrations are determined in part by activity of the P_{450} isozymes that catalyze the hydroxylation and demethylation of the TCAs, and both genetics and environment may alter activity of these enzymes.

In the 1960s, Alexanderson and colleagues (1969) demonstrated the importance of both genetic and environmental factors on TCA metabolism. Studying twin pairs, these authors found that for those twins who were not concomitantly taking any other medications, monozygotic twins achieved similar steady-state NT concentrations, and dizygotic twins did not. However, for those monozygotic twins who were taking other medications, this intrapair similarity in steady-state concentrations was not found. Alexanderson (1972) went on to demonstrate that, within individuals, plasma concentrations and clearance rates of the secondary amine TCAs NT and DMI correlated, suggesting that plasma kinetics of these two TCAs are "regulated by common genetic factors" (p. 8). Hammer and Sjoqvist (1967) made similar observations about NT and DMI plasma concentrations.

To further assess the effects of genetics and environment of the metabolism of TCAs, researchers have looked for probes of the various metabolic steps such as hydroxylation and demethylation that may be influenced by genetic and environmental factors. Several investigators have linked TCA metabolism to the 4-hydroxylation of the antihypertensive debrisoquine by a specific P_{450} isozyme. In single-dose studies of volunteer subjects, hydroxylation clearance of NT (Bertilsson et al. 1980; Mellstrom et al. 1981; Woolhouse et al. 1984), hydroxylation of IMI (Skjelbo et al. 1991), hydroxylation of clomipramine (Balant-Gorgia et al. 1986), and hydroxylation of DMI (Spina et al. 1984) were all found to correlate with debrisoquine hydroxylation. These findings were supported by in vitro studies of human liver microsomes (Brosen et al. 1991; Spina et al. 1984; von Bahr et al. 1983, 1986). Steady-state concentrations of NT (Nordin et al. 1985) and DMI (Bertilsson and Aberg-Wistedt 1983) in depressed patients were also found to correlate with debrisoquine hydroxylation.

The activity of the debrisoquine hydroxylase isozyme varies

between individuals, with cross-ethnic differences existing in the frequency of PM (poor metabolizer [or poor metabolizing]) phenotype (see Table 2–3 and Chapter 2 for discussion). Some have reported that PM of debrisoquine correlates with diminished metabolism of TCAs, leading to higher TCA concentrations for a given dose. If this is true, decreased metabolism of TCAs should occur more frequently in Caucasians, as they display a greater frequency of PM of debrisoquine. Interestingly, Caucasians are members of the one racial or ethnic group that has not been linked clinically to decreased TCA metabolism. This inconsistency may be related to several factors.

First, the impact of PM of debrisoquine on TCA metabolism depends on the relative contribution of hydroxylation clearance to overall clearance of the agent. As TCAs undergo other metabolic steps, including demethylation and conjugation, the relative contribution of hydroxylation is less than with an agent whose only metabolic step is hydroxylation. TCA demethylation has not been shown to correlate with debrisoquine hydroxylation (Mellstrom et al. 1983; von Bahr et al. 1986). Balant-Gorgia and colleagues (1982) found that although AT hydroxylation correlates with debrisoquine hydroxylation, steady-state AT is more dependent on demethylation. Second, both the isozyme involved in debrisoquine hydroxylation and other isozymes involved in TCA metabolism may be induced or inhibited by environmental factors. Third, as described in Chapter 2, the average activity of debrisoquine hydroxylase in Caucasian patients who are extensive metabolizers (EMs) is higher than in Asian and African patients who are EMs (Kalow 1991).

When studied as a probe of hepatic activity, the hydroxylation of S-mephenytoin, the hydantoin anticonvulsant displays different phenotypy than debrisoquine (Bertilsson et al. 1989; Nakamura et al. 1985); yet, like debrisoquine, it shows variation between different ethnic groups (see Chapter 2 and Table 2–4). Demethylation of the TCA IMI has recently been shown by one study (Skjelbo et al. 1991) to correlate highly with hydroxylation of S-mephenytoin. Thus, ethnic differences in the activity of this isozyme may contribute to ethnic variations in metabolism of TCAs—particularly the tertiary amines, as demethylation is a significant step in their metabolism.

PHARMACODYNAMICS OF TCAs

TCAs are believed to exert their antidepressant response indirectly through effects on receptors, and it is possible that these receptor effects may also vary between people of different ethnic backgrounds. Differences in the pharmacodynamics have been clearly demonstrated with regard to the effects of certain non-psychiatric medications such as propranolol (Kalow 1989; Zhou et al. 1989) and have been suggested to be a contributing factor in differences in ethnic responses to the antipsychotic haloperidol (Lin and Poland 1989). Although this issue has not been directly examined with regard to TCAs, evidence suggests that ethnic differences in therapeutic plasma concentrations (Hu et al. 1983; Yamashita and Asano 1979) and sensitivity to emergent side effects from TCAs exist, as will be discussed in the next section.

CLINICAL IMPRESSIONS REGARDING PHARMACOLOGY AND ETHNICITY

Multinational Study

In 1986, a World Health Organization Collaborative Study compared "low-dose" (37.5–56 mg/day) and "high-dose" (75.0–150.0 mg/day) treatment of depression with AT, maprotiline (MAP), or IMI in several countries. Patients with various depressive diagnoses were monitored and treatment response was measured by rating scales. The study reported that the patients receiving "higher dosages" responded better, but not to a significant degree. When dosages were freely adjusted at the individual centers, the researchers found that the average daily dose was lowered slightly from the initial fixed dose in Switzerland; Bombay, India; Colombia; and Japan, and raised slightly from the initial fixed dose in Lucknow, India, and the United States. Information on the ethnic backgrounds of the patients in the United States was not available. Although patients in the United States might be considered to need higher doses of TCAs than patients in the other countries, few additional conclusions can be drawn from this study. The "high-dose" regimen was a modest one and could be considered subtherapeutic. In addition, TCA concentrations were not available, rendering the interpretation of the results of this study difficult.

Studies of East Asians

Of the various ethnic groups studied with regard to differences in prescribing practices, clinical efficacy, and side effects of TCAs, the most extensively studied is the East Asian population. In the 1970s, Yamashita and Asano (1979) examined TCA-prescribing practices in Asia. They reported that the doses of the tertiary amines AT and IMI prescribed in Asian countries, 70–134 mg/day, were much lower than the doses prescribed in the United States. The data used in making this observation came from a survey of psychiatrists in 10 East Asian countries who were treating patients for endogenous depression. Yamashita and Asano also provided data from their own longitudinal evaluation of steady-state plasma TCA concentrations in patients treated successfully for depression, including 22 patients treated with IMI and 26 patients treated with AT. They found that TCA concentrations were not particularly high in relation to dosage administered, suggesting that Asians do not necessarily metabolize TCAs differently than Caucasians do and that depressed Asian patients may respond to fairly low steady-state concentrations of TCAs.

In 1981, Kleinman reported his observations regarding the treatment of major depression in Chinese in the People's Republic of China with TCAs including doxepin (DOX), IMI, and AT. He observed that the "therapeutic threshold dose" of these medications needed for Chinese subjects was 75 mg/day (as compared to 150 mg/day needed for most Caucasians) and that most of the Chinese patients responded to a daily dose of 100 mg. These findings are in agreement with those of Yamashita and Asano (1979) that Chinese may respond to lower TCA dosages.

In the early 1980s, clinicians and researchers working with Asians in the United States began to turn their attention to the diagnosis and treatment of psychiatric disorders in this group. Kinzie and Manson (1983) reported on 5 years' experience working in a specialized Indochinese Psychiatric Clinic in Oregon. They found a higher percentage of Asian patients (48%) with a major affective disorder, as compared to 28% of patients attending a general adult outpatient psychiatric clinic at their institution. Similar to Yamashita and Asano (1979) as well as Kleinman (1981), they found that the highest average TCA dose that was prescribed for this cohort (110 mg of IMI or its equivalent) was lower than that prescribed for a comparable Western population treated for severe depression.

Rosenblat and Tang (1987) reviewed charts of 33 Asian patients and 33 matched Caucasians, all living in Canada, some of whom were treated with AT. As in the three studies cited previously, in examining the doses prescribed relative to body weight, the authors found that the maximal doses of AT prescribed for Asians were significantly lower than those prescribed for their Caucasian counterparts.

Studies of African-Americans

Although they were not studied as extensively as Asians, the earliest observations that demonstrated race may be a factor in determining clinical response occurred in a study comparing African-Americans and Caucasians. In a multicenter Veterans Administration study of patients treated with TCAs, including AT and NT, Overall and colleagues (1969) found that African-American patients improved more rapidly than Caucasian patients. Similarly, in a clinical study of outpatients in a university psychiatric clinic who had mixed symptoms of depression and anxiety, Henry and colleagues (1971) rated subject responses to TCAs alone, TCAs in conjunction with benzodiazepines, or benzodiazepines alone. The authors found that African-American and Hispanic patients responded better to pharmacotherapy as compared to Caucasian patients. This finding held for treatment with TCAs, but even more strongly for treatment with benzodiazepines. As this study did not compare drug treatment with placebo treatment, placebo response cannot be ruled out as a confounding factor.

In 1975, Raskin and Crook reported on a multihospital collaborative study of the differential effects of chlorpromazine and IMI in African-American and Caucasian inpatients with symptoms (but not necessarily a diagnosis) of depression. Patients were assigned to treatment with IMI, chlorpromazine, or placebo in a double-blind manner, and treatment response was measured with several rating scales. This study, like that of Overall and colleagues (1969), found that African-American patients improved more rapidly than did Caucasian patients. African-American men were more responsive to IMI and African-American women were more responsive to chlorpromazine. Interpretations of this study are confounded by the study design, which included patients with varying diagnoses (i.e., schizophrenia, involutional psychotic reaction, psychotic depression, and simple depression) being treated with IMI (a TCA) or chlorpromazine (an antipsychotic). In addition, the two ethnic groups were not similar in age, the average age of the African-Americans being approximately 10 years younger than that of the Caucasians.

Studies of Hispanics

A collaborative study in mental health clinics in the United States (Adams et al. 1984) examined diagnosis and pharmacotherapy in Hispanics as compared with African-Americans and Caucasians. Adams and colleagues found that Hispanics were prescribed psychotropic medications less frequently, but when they *were* prescribed medications, they were prescribed similar numbers of medications as the other groups. No data are available on the dosages of TCAs prescribed to the various groups.

Escobar and Tuason (1980) reported on treatment of 40 patients in Colombia and 32 patients in the United States, all of whom had been diagnosed with either unipolar or bipolar depression. Response to trazodone was compared with response to both IMI and placebo as measured by reduction in Hamilton Rating Scale for Depression (HAM-D; Hamilton 1960) score. They found IMI but not trazodone to be superior to placebo in both countries. The patients in Colombia improved more than those in the United States regardless of treatment, with a high percentage of the Colombian group responding to placebo. Also, more Colombians reported anticholinergic side effects when treated with IMI. Although this study indicates possible differences in the response to antidepressants between the patients in the United States and those in Colombia, conclusions cannot be drawn with regard to ethnic variations; the majority of patients in both countries were Caucasians, with a few African-Americans participating. Study design is also problematic, as initially the Colombian patients displayed more severe symptoms than those in the United States and the average age of the Colombian group was 6 years older than that of the United States group.

In a review of outpatient pharmacotherapy of major depression, Marcos and Cancro (1982) compared the dosages of various TCAs (AT, IMI, or DOX) used to treat 41 Hispanic females (primarily Puerto Ricans) with the dosages used to treat 21 Caucasian females. All patients were free of medical illness and were not taking any other medications. The authors found that the mean maximum daily dosage of the Hispanic group (64 mg/day) was only about one-half of the mean maximum daily dosage of the Caucasian group (130 mg/day). Yet a higher percentage of the Hispanic patients complained of side effects (78% versus 33%)—a finding which the authors ascribe to the Hispanic tradition of expressing depression in somatic terms. In addition, despite the lower dosages prescribed for Hispanic patients, the two groups had very similar treatment outcomes, with 75.6% of the Hispanics and 71.4% of the Caucasians "improving." Comparison of these groups is limited by differences in age (with the Hispanics an average of 10 years younger than the Caucasians) and lack of control of consumption of alcohol and use of tobacco, although patients were eliminated from both groups if they were taking any other medications. No data were available on TCA concentrations; thus, it is impossible to ascertain whether the differences found with regard to dosage and side effects were related to TCA pharmacokinetics.

KINETIC STUDIES IN CONTROL SUBJECTS

Beginning in the late 1970s, there have been several attempts to use kinetic studies in control subjects to clarify issues of possible interethnic differences in TCA metabolism. These studies unfortunately have yielded somewhat inconsistent results (see Table 4–1). Most of the literature in this field deals with Asians, possibly because they collectively represent more than one-half of the world population (United Nations 1988).

Table 4–1. Kinetic studies in volunteer control subjects

Authors	Volunteers studied	TCA dose	Assay method	Findings
Allen et al. 1977	6 Asian Indians 11 British Caucasians males all in England	CMI 25 and 50 mg CMI 25 and 50 mg		Greater S/E, AUC, higher peak [CMI] in Asian Indians
Lewis et al. 1980	14 British in England	CMI 25 and 50 mg		No change from previous findings
Kishimoto and Hollister 1984	10 Japanese in Japan 10 Caucasians in United States males	NT 50 mg	GLC electron capture	Higher peak [NT], greater AUC in Japanese
Schneider et al. 1991	Asians 8 Caucasians	NT 40 mg		Greater AUC NT and 10-OH NT, 1990 decreased CL_{NT} in Asians
Rudorfer et al. 1984	14 Chinese 16 Caucasians sex-matched	DMI 100 mg	HPLC	Higher peak and mean [DMI], earlier peak DMI, decreased CL_{DMI} in Chinese, trimodal dist of CL_{DMI}
Pi et al. 1986	9 Chinese 3 Koreans 8 Japanese 20 Caucasians[a]	DMI 50 mg DMI 50 mg DMI 50 mg DMI 75 mg	GC	Peak [DMI] earlier in Asians
Pi et al. 1989	7 Chinese 2 Japanese 9 Vietnamese 19 Caucasians age-matched	DMI 1mg/kg	HPLC	Peak [DMI] earlier in Caucasians, C_{IDMI} and CL_{OHDMI} greater in Caucasians (prior to wt correction), CL_{DMI} and CL_{OHDMI} trimodal in all
Gaviria et al. 1986	10 Hispanics 10 Caucasians	NT 75 mg NT 75 mg	GLC	No significant pharmacokinetic differences

Note. AUC = area under the curve; CMI = clomipramine; DMI = desipramine; GLC = gas-liquid chromatography; NT = nortriptyline; S/E = side effects.
[a] Indicates Caucasians were studied previously and used for comparison.

Although kinetic studies in volunteer subjects provide valuable information regarding the fate of medications in human bodies, for several reasons, caution must be exercised in extending findings of these studies into clinical situations. First, the kinetic profile of patients may be altered by the disease process and thus may not correspond well to findings based on control subject studies. In addition, despite reports of high correlation between single-dose kinetics and steady-state drug levels, the two are not necessarily identical, and it is these steady-state levels that determine clinical response (Asberg et al. 1970, 1971; Sjoqvist et al. 1971). Finally, these studies cannot provide any data pertaining to clinical response to medications.

Studies of Asian Indians

Allen and colleagues (1977) completed one of the earliest pharmacokinetic studies in volunteer subjects, comparing side effect profiles and plasma concentrations after 25- or 50-mg single doses of the tertiary amine clomipramine (CMI) in British and Asian Indian (Pakistani and Indian) volunteer subjects in England. Preliminary data on 11 British subjects (unknown ethnicity) and 6 Asian Indian male subjects indicated that the incidence and severity of self-reported side effects appeared to be greater among the Asian Indians and that this group also attained higher peak plasma CMI concentrations. The higher peak concentrations in Asians reached statistical significance only after the 50-mg dosage (45.1 ng/ml versus 25.7 ng/ml). In 1980, Lewis and colleagues reported data obtained on 14 additional British volunteer subjects, indicating a persistence of the pattern of greater side effects and higher peak levels in the Asian Indian subjects. Calculation of the area under the curve (AUC), an indication of the total amount of drug present in the plasma over a given period, also indicated a significant difference after the 50-mg dosage, with the AUC being greater for the Asian Indians.

Studies of East Asians

Kishimoto and Hollister (1984) compared single-dose NT kinetics in 10 male Japanese volunteer subjects (ages 22–25 living in Japan) to 10 Caucasian males (ages 22–30 living in the United

States). Volunteer subjects who used alcohol or street drugs or who were heavy users of tobacco were excluded from the study. The Japanese were given 50 mg of powdered NT, and the Caucasians were given 100 mg of powdered NT. Plasma NT assays were performed independently in the two countries by gas-liquid chromatography (GLC)–electron capture. Despite having taken only one-half the dose taken by the Caucasians, the Japanese achieved slightly higher peak plasma NT concentrations. The AUC was also significantly higher in the Japanese subjects (1,150 ng/ml/hour compared to 730 ng/ml/hour). No differences were found between the two groups with regard to NT half-life ($t_{1/2}$) or time to peak plasma concentration.

Schneider and colleagues (1991) more recently performed a pilot study of NT kinetics in six Asians (subgroup unknown) and eight Caucasians, who were similar in age and body weight. A dose of 40 mg of NT was administered to each of the subjects. As with Kishimoto and Hollister (1984), the authors found a trend for increased bioavailability of NT in the Asians, with the AUC of the Asians (1,509 ng/ml/hour) being greater than that of the Caucasians (920 ng/ml/hour). In addition, Schneider and colleagues found increased bioavailability of 10-hydroxy-NT as well as decreased clearance of NT in the Asian group. Although this study was based on a very small sample size, they postulated a relatively reduced rate of hepatic hydroxylation in Asians compared to Caucasians, as well as possibly a different handling of 10-hydroxy-NT.

Rudorfer and colleagues (1984) investigated DMI kinetics in 14 Chinese and 16 Caucasian volunteer subjects, all in the United States. Study participants were screened for use of routine medications and "excessive" alcohol use, but smokers were not excluded from participation. A dose of 100 mg of DMI was administered to each subject, followed by a 4-day period of blood collection and a 5-day period of urine collection. Plasma and urine concentrations of DMI and 2-hydroxy-DMI were measured by high-performance liquid chromatography (HPLC). The authors found that the Chinese manifested higher mean peak DMI concentrations (45.4 ng/ml versus 29.8 ng/ml) and mean peak 2-hydroxy-DMI concentrations (28.0 ng/ml versus 20.6 ng/ml) than the Caucasians, and that the mean DMI concentrations of the Chinese remained higher than those of the Caucasians throughout the trial. In addition, the mean clearance of DMI (CL_{DMI}) was significantly lower in the Chinese than the Caucasians. A trimodal distribution was found for CL_{DMI}, not associated with body weight, with Chinese primarily evidencing "slow" clearance and Caucasians primarily showing "rapid" clearance, indicating that some Chinese may be at risk for toxicity. They did not find significant differences in DMI elimination ($t_{1/2}$), clearance of DMI to 2-hydroxy-DMI, or the fraction of DMI bound to plasma protein. Rudorfer and colleagues concluded that Chinese volunteer subjects metabolize DMI more slowly than Caucasians, and that this metabolic difference accounts for lower dosage requirements by Chinese.

Rudorfer and colleagues (1985) subsequently attempted to correlate debrisoquine hydroxylation with CL_{DMI} in 10 of the 16 Caucasians and 9 of the 14 Chinese subjects, along with 1 additional Chinese woman. After single doses of debrisoquine 10 mg, urinary concentrations of debrisoquine and its 10-hydroxymetabolite were measured by gas chromatography (GC)–electron capture. None of these 20 subjects were poor metabolizers of debrisoquine, and thus slow CL_{DMI} as found in the volunteer subjects in the first study could not be correlated with poor metabolism of debrisoquine. As stated earlier, metabolism of DMI is more complex than that of debrisoquine, possibly accounting for this discrepancy. In addition, the small sample size makes conclusions preliminary.

Pi and colleagues (1986) also completed a study of DMI kinetics in the United States. Twenty Asian volunteer subjects, both male and female, were studied. The 20 subjects included 9 Chinese, 8 Japanese, and 3 Koreans, each of whom was given 50 mg of DMI. Plasma DMI assays were performed by GC, and the pharmacokinetic parameters were compared with parameters generated in a previous study of 20 Caucasians who had been given DMI 75 mg. The only significant pharmacokinetic difference that was found between the two groups was that plasma DMI concentration peaked earlier in the Asians. The remainder of the pharmacokinetic parameters, including peak serum DMI concentration, V_d, plasma clearance, elimination $t_{1/2}$, and peak DMI concentration normalized to 1 mg/kg, were not significantly different between the Asians and the Caucasians. The authors appropriately comment that as within each ethnic group the parameters studied showed large variation, it would be difficult to discern whether or not significant pharmacokinetic differences exist between the ethnic groups. In addition, the heterogeneity of the Asian group makes specific ethnic comparisons impossible.

In 1989, Pi and colleagues published a more sophisticated study of single-dose DMI kinetics, involving 18 Asian and 19 Caucasian volunteer subjects. The Asian group included 11 males and 7 females, with 9 Vietnamese, 7 Chinese, and 2 Japanese subjects, with an average age of 28.7 years. The Caucasian group included 12 males and 7 females, with an average age of 31.8 years. Each subject was given DMI 1.0 mg/kg, and plasma samples were assayed by HPLC for DMI and 2-hydroxy-DMI. In contrast to the findings in their previous study in which DMI concentrations peaked earlier in Asians, the authors found in this second study that plasma DMI concentrations actually peaked later in the Asians (5 hours versus 3 hours in Caucasians). Consistent with their previous study, however, they found no significant difference in other parameters, including peak plasma DMI concentration or elimination $t_{1/2}$. The additional parameters studied, CL_{DMI} and 2-hydroxy-DMI, were greater in Caucasians only prior to correction for the greater body weight of the Caucasians. Also, the fraction of DMI metabolized to 2-hydroxy-DMI and the fraction of DMI excreted unchanged were not significantly different between the groups. The data on fractional metabolism of DMI to 2-hydroxy-DMI showed slow, intermediate, and fast metabolizers in both ethnic groups, with more Caucasians being rapid metabolizers, consistent with the findings of Rudorfer and colleagues (1984). As with their previous study, this study suffers from ethnic heterogeneity in the Asian group, as well as large variations in the pharmacokinetic data in each ethnic group.

Studies of Hispanics

Gaviria and colleagues (1986) published the only study of TCA pharmacokinetics in Hispanic volunteer subjects, comparing NT kinetics in the Hispanics with those in age-, sex-, and weight-matched Caucasian volunteer subjects, all of whom were free from tobacco use, alcohol abuse, medical or psychiatric illness, or other pharmacotherapy. Plasma samples drawn from each of the volunteer subjects after single doses of 75 mg of NT were analyzed by GLC. Pharmacokinetic parameters, including absorption $t_{1/2}$, elimination $t_{1/2}$, AUC, V_d, total clearance (CL), C_{max}, and T_{max}, showed no significant differences between the Hispanic and the Caucasian subjects, nor between the male and female subgroups within each ethnic group. However, as in the studies by Pi and colleagues (1986, 1989), great variation was found in these parameters among the individuals in this study. Gaviria and colleagues concluded that pharmacokinetic factors may not be responsible for previous clinical findings suggesting a lower therapeutic dose range and more side effects in Hispanics than in Caucasians. They postulated that ethnic differences may exist due to variables not studied here, such as receptor binding, or the effect of the disease of depression on pharmacokinetics.

CLINICAL STUDIES

Studies of East Asians

Hu and colleagues (1983) examined TCA concentrations in severely depressed hospitalized Chinese patients receiving fixed doses of IMI (150 mg/day). They found that the minimal combined therapeutic IMI and DMI concentration was 130 ng/ml, a concentration lower than had been previously reported in American and European studies (the 1985 APA Task Force on the Use of Laboratory Tests in Psychiatry), indicating that Chinese subjects may respond to lower concentrations of TCAs, similar to the earlier findings of Yamashita and Asano (1979) for Japanese subjects.

Kinzie and colleagues (1987) studied TCA blood concentrations in three distinct groups of Asian outpatients in the United States who were on long-term TCA therapy. A total of 41 Vietnamese, Cambodian, and Mien patients undergoing IMI therapy were monitored, with IMI and DMI concentrations measured by HPLC. The authors initially found a high rate of noncompliance, particularly among the Vietnamese and Mien subjects (as judged by 61% of the patients having no detectable TCA concentrations). After the patients were educated about the medications, the noncompliance rate fell to 37%. Kinzie and colleagues went on to present preliminary data on 19 patients who were judged to be compliant, based on description of side effects and, in some cases, pill count. In contrast to the findings of Hu (1983), Kinzie and colleagues stated that the data collected from this second group indicate that "Asians generally need doses of tricyclics similar to those required by Caucasians" (p. 484) to attain a TCA level greater than 180 ng/ml. However, the authors stated that a small group of patients developed therapeutic concentrations on lower dosages, but extension of these conclusions is limited by the small sample size and the inclusion of Vietnamese, Cambodian, and Mien in the Asian group.

In related research, one of us (B. A. Silver, S. Potkin, unpublished data, November 1992) retrospectively compared NT dosage and blood concentrations in 10 Vietnamese patients to those of 10 age- and sex-matched Caucasians. Data on smoking were not recorded, but patients were excluded from the review if they were taking any medications that were known to influence serum TCA concentrations. The Vietnamese were prescribed, on the average, lower NT dosages than the Caucasians (70 mg/day versus 103 mg/day). Yet when dosage given was calculated on a mg/kg body weight basis to account for the lower average body weight of the Asians, the dosages prescribed to the two groups were not significantly different (1.49 mg/kg for the Vietnamese and 1.65 mg/kg for the Caucasians). No significant difference was found between the groups with regard to average plasma NT concentration (92 ng/ml for the Vietnamese and 111 ng/ml for the Caucasians). As with previous studies, conclusions are limited by the small sample size and the retrospective nature of the study.

We prospectively examined DMI treatment of major depression in 52 patients, including 22 Caucasians and 30 Asians (including 18 Vietnamese, 5 Chinese, 6 Japanese, and 1 Pilipino). Preliminary analysis revealed that although the mean steady-state relative serum DMI concentrations (serum DMI concentrations divided by daily doses) were similar among Caucasians,

Chinese, and Japanese subjects, the Vietnamese patients had significantly higher steady-state relative DMI concentrations. Moreover, this difference remained significant after controlling for the lower mean body weight of the Vietnamese subjects.

Studies of African-Americans

Ziegler and Biggs (1977) examined steady-state plasma TCA concentrations in a total of 65 Caucasian and African-American depressed patients, 35 of whom were treated with AT and 30 of whom were treated with NT, without any concomitant drug therapy. GC-mass fragmentography was used to determine TCA concentrations. The authors corrected for individual doses so that individual patient's plasma concentrations were based on a 1 mg/kg oral dose. Plasma TCA concentrations varied tenfold in AT-treated patients. Among the AT treated patients, the African patients had 27% higher average TCA concentrations than the Caucasians, but this did not reach statistical significance, and there was not a significant difference in the rate of demethylation of AT to NT between the two groups. Among the NT treated patients, the African-American patients had significantly (50%) higher NT concentrations than the Caucasian patients. The authors conclude that the higher NT plasma concentrations found in African-Americans may produce a more rapid response to TCA treatment such as was described by Overall and colleagues (1969).

Plasma TCA concentrations in Caucasian and African-American patients being treated after AT overdose were examined retrospectively by Rudorfer and Robins (1982). Of the 24 patients studied, 5 were Caucasian males, 13 were Caucasian females, and 6 were African-American females. The authors found a correlation between amount of AT ingested reportedly ingested and total TCA concentration as measured by GLC-mass spectrophotometry. In examining the two ethnic groups, a 30% higher mean plasma TCA concentration was found in the African-American patients as compared with the Caucasian patients, yet these values were not significantly different from each other. After calculating plasma TCA concentration per milligram AT reportedly ingested, they found that African-Americans, on the average, generated a plasma TCA concentration to dose ratio twice as high as found in the Caucasians. The ratio of AT to NT was also slightly, but not significantly, greater in the African-Americans, possibly indicating slower demethylation by African-Americans. However, it is important to note that plasma was also obtained slightly earlier from the African-Americans than from the Caucasians (5.2 hours versus 6.8 hours) allowing less time for demethylation to occur. This study suggests, as does the previous study by Ziegler and Biggs, that African-Americans may develop higher TCA concentrations than Caucasians with similar doses of TCAs.

An indirect comparison of TCA effects in Caucasian and African-American patients was performed by Livingston and colleagues (1983). This study reported on a review of charts of 125 inpatients who were being treated with TCAs and had plasma TCA determinations. The authors sought to identify risk factors for the development of delirium during the course of TCA treatment, and they found that age, race, and log plasma TCA concentration "contributed equally and independently to the occurrence of delirium" (p. 174). Although only 5 of the 102 Caucasian patients (4.9%) reportedly met DSM-III (American Psychiatric Association 1980) criteria for delirium, 5 of the 23 African-American patients (21.7%) met these same criteria. The average plasma TCA concentration was 321 ng/ml for the patients who developed delirium but was only 125 ng/ml for the entire group of patients. The authors cite possible anticholinergic toxicity due to elevated TCA concentrations as a possible etiology for delirium, yet in 9 of the 10 patients, signs of peripheral anticholinergic toxicity were absent. It is possible that race and TCA concentration are independently related to the development of delirium and that pharmacodynamic factors such as receptor sensitivity might underlie the greater susceptibility to delirium in African-Americans undergoing therapy with TCAs.

Studies of Saudi Arabians

The only known clinical study of TCA concentrations in Saudi Arabian patients was performed by El-Yazigi and Chaleby (1988). Twenty-one Saudi patients were maintained on DOX (average dose 50 mg/day), and 30 were maintained on IMI (average dose 100 mg/day). Plasma samples were analyzed by HPLC and concentrations were compared with those previously reported for Western patients. The authors corrected steady-state TCA concentrations to be based on a mg/kg dose. The DOX-treated Saudi patients demonstrated a mean dose-normalized steady-state DOX concentration greater than values reported for Western patients. The IMI-treated patients also displayed higher dose normalized steady-state TCA concentrations than were reported in three out of four studies on Western patients. The calculated mean ratio of the steady-state concentration of DMI to that of IMI was lower in the Saudis than ratios in American or European subjects, indicating that Saudis either demethylate IMI more slowly or eliminate DMI more rapidly than Americans or Europeans. The authors comment that more rapid elimination of desipramine may be related to the lower frequency of debrisoquine PM found among Saudis than among Caucasian Britons (Islam et al. 1980).

CONCLUSIONS

The study of the psychopharmacology of ethnicity is complex, encompassing many variables, including clinical practice and genetic, environmental, and cultural issues. Studies addressing the questions of clinical efficacy and side effects of TCAs in different ethnic groups must take all of these variables into account.

Asian Indians. Limited pharmacokinetic data suggest that, compared with Caucasians, Asian Indian volunteer subjects may attain higher plasma concentrations and report more side effects than Caucasians after single doses of the tertiary amine CMI. Generalizations regarding the clinical efficacy and therapeutic concentrations of TCAs or the metabolism of secondary amines in depressed Asian Indians are not available.

East Asians. Several authors have found that depression in the Asian patients may possibly be treated with dosages of tertiary amine TCAs that are lower than are customarily used to treat depression in Caucasian patients (Kinzie and Manson 1983; Kleinman 1981; Rosenblat and Tang 1987; Yamashita and Asano 1979). Several kinetic studies have attempted to elicit whether these lower doses might produce higher plasma concentrations in Asians than in Caucasians. Both Kishimoto and Hollister (1984), studying the Japanese, and Schneider and colleagues (1991), studying a mix of Asian subgroups, found that Asians metabolize NT more slowly than Caucasians, and Rudorfer and colleagues (1984) found a similar tendency for Chinese subjects with the DMI. Rudorfer and colleagues also found trimodal clearance patterns, with more of the Asians evidencing slow clearance.

In contrast to these findings, Pi and colleagues (1986, 1989) did not find significant differences in DMI kinetics when comparing Chinese, Japanese, and Koreans with Caucasians. Like Rudorfer and colleagues (1984), Pi and colleagues (1989) found that slightly more Asians could be classified as "slow metabolizers." The confounding findings of these kinetic studies are likely related not only to small sample sizes, but to the inclusion of separate Asian subgroups in statistical calculations. The literature regarding steady-state blood concentrations and the clinical response of depressed Asians to TCAs is also not entirely consistent. In Taiwan, Hu and colleagues (1983) found that Asians may respond to lower therapeutic concentrations of TCAs than Caucasians. However, in the United States, Kinzie and Manson (1983) found that a mixed group of Asians may need doses of TCAs similar to those received by Caucasians to obtain adequate blood levels. In research also conducted by one of us in the United States, it was found that NT doses expressed as mg/kg body weight taken by 10 Vietnamese patients were similar to those taken by 10 Caucasian patients, and NT plasma concentrations were also comparable between the two races (B. A. Silver, S. Potkin, unpublished data, November 1992). However, higher steady-state DMI concentrations were found in a group of Vietnamese patients as compared to Caucasians, Japanese, and Chinese.

African-Americans. Initial clinical impressions suggested that African-Americans may respond both better and more rapidly to TCAs than Caucasians. Three clinical studies have suggested that this response may be due to higher TCA concentrations achieved in African-Americans as compared to Caucasians. Ziegler and Biggs (1977) found that African-American patients developed higher TCA concentrations than Caucasians per milligram of AT or NT ingested. Similarly, African-American patients who overdosed on AT had significantly higher TCA concentrations than their Caucasian counterparts, and slightly higher AT/NT ratios (Rudorfer and Robins 1982). Another study (Livingston et al. 1983) indicated that a higher percentage of African-American patients being treated with TCAs developed delirium during the course of treatment than did Caucasian patients. Without any data from kinetic studies in patients or control subjects, it is impossible to ascertain with certainty whether the greater response to TCAs seen in African-Americans is entirely due to metabolic differences.

Hispanics. The paucity of literature regarding the use of TCAs in Hispanic patients has suggested both improvement and greater side effects at lower dosages (Marcos and Cancro 1982) and greater response to both placebo and TCAs among Hispanics as compared to their Caucasian counterparts. One study with NT (Gaviria et al. 1986), demonstrating a lack of kinetic variation between Hispanics and Caucasians, indicated that if Hispanics do respond more favorably to lower dosages this response may be due to pharmacodynamic differences.

Saudi Arabians. A limited clinical study indicates that during treatment with both IMI and DOX, Saudi Arabians may develop higher mean dose-normalized steady-state TCA levels than Western patients. In addition, the Saudi patients either demethylate IMI more slowly or eliminate DMI more rapidly than Caucasians, as indicated by lower ratios of DMI to IMI at steady state.

FUTURE DIRECTIONS

Further clarification of the questions regarding the metabolism, pharmacodynamics, side effects, and clinical efficacy of TCAs in different ethnic groups is necessary. Studies have indicated that it is possible that black Africans, Asians, and Hispanics may respond to lower dosages and/or concentrations of TCAs than Caucasians, and yet the precise nature of these variations remains unclear. Thus far, the majority of studies have focused on Asian populations. Yet even these studies are not completely conclusive, with broadly defined groups of Asians in variable environmental settings being included in the same study. Studies that have larger sample sizes and compare specific ethnic groups with similar environmental exposures and concurrent pharmacologic interventions must be performed. Consistency in TCA assay location is also critical, as a survey of laboratories involved in TCA assays indicated a high coefficient of variation (30%) among the laboratories (Task Force on the Use of Laboratory Tests in Psychiatry 1985).

As several studies indicate that debrisoquine/sparteine hydroxylation status influences TCA metabolism (Bertilsson and Aberg-Wistedt 1983; Bertilsson et al. 1980; Mellstrom et al. 1981; Nordin et al. 1985; Skjelbo et al. 1991; Spina et al. 1984; Woolhouse et al. 1984), and one study indicates that mephenytoin hydroxylation status correlates with IMI demethylation (Skjelbo et al. 1991), interethnic studies of phenotypic status in relationship to TCA metabolism and response may assist in answering questions about pharmacokinetic contributions to ethnic differences in TCA administration and response.

Another important yet unanswered question is that of interethnic variations in the interaction of TCAs with other agents, as most reports on drug interactions are related to experience with Caucasians. A critical example of this is the elevation of TCA levels when TCAs are combined with fluoxetine, as fluoxetine is widely used by both psychiatrists and nonpsychiatrists. Suggestions that this interaction may be due to inhibition of debrisoquine hydroxylase by fluoxetine and norfluoxetine may indicate that ethnic groups such as Asians and black Africans who have low levels of debrisoquine hydroxylase activity may be at higher risk for developing dangerous TCA toxicities when treated with these two agents.

In addition, there is little knowledge of any interethnic differences that may exist with regard to metabolism and response of various ethnic groups to the newer antidepressants, such as fluoxetine, buproprion, and sertraline. Future research mandates not only resolution of the questions of interethnic variation with regard to the TCAs but also to these new antidepressants as well.

REFERENCES

Adams GL, Dworkin RJ, Rosenberg SD: Diagnosis and pharmacotherapy issues in the care of Hispanics in the public sector. Am J Psychiatry 141:970–974, 1984

Alexanderson B: Pharmacokinetics of desmethylimipramine and nortriptyline and man after single and multiple oral doses—a cross-over study. Eur J Clin Pharmacol 5:1–10, 1972

Alexanderson B, Borga O: Interindividual differences in plasma protein binding of nortriptyline in man: a twin study. Eur J Clin Pharmacol 4:196–200, 1972

Alexanderson B, Price-Evans DA, Sjoqvist F: Steady-state plasma levels of nortriptyline in twins: influence of genetic factors and drug therapy. BMJ 4:764–768, 1969

Allen JJ, Vaddadi KS, Rack PH: Differences in the effects of clomipramine on English and Asian volunteers: preliminary report on a pilot study. Postgrad Med J 53 (suppl 4):79–86, 1977

American Psychiatric Association: Diagnostic and Statistical Manual of Mental Disorders, 3rd Edition. Washington, DC, American Psychiatric Association, 1980

Asberg M, Cronholm B, Sjoqvist F, et al: Correlation of subjective side effects with plasma concentrations of nortriptyline. BMJ 4:18–21, 1970

Asberg M, Cronholm B, Sjoqvist F, et al: Relationship between plasma level and therapeutic effect of nortriptyline. BMJ 3:331–334, 1971

Balant-Gorgia AE, Schultz P, Dayer P, et al: Role of oxidation polymorphism on blood and urine concentrations of amitriptyline and its metabolites in man. Arch Psychiatr Nervenkr 232:215–222, 1982

Balant-Gorgia AE, Balant LP, Genet C, et al: Importance of oxidative polymorphism and levopromazine treatment of the steady-state concentrations of clomipramine and its major metabolites. Eur J Clin Pharmacol 31:449–455, 1986

Balderassini RJ: Chemotherapy in Psychiatry: Principles and Practice. Cambridge, MA, Harvard University Press, 1985

Bertilsson L, Aberg-Wistedt A: The debrisoquine hydroxylation test predicts steady-state plasma levels of desipramine. Br J Clin Pharmacol 15:388–390, 1983

Bertilsson L, Eichelbaum M, Mellstrom B, et al: Nortriptyline and antipyrine clearance in relation to debrisoquine hydroxylation in man. Life Sci 27:1673–1677, 1980

Bertilsson L, Henthorn TK, Sanz E, et al: Importance of genetic factors in the regulation of diazepam metabolism: relationship to S-mephenytoin, but not debrisoquine phenotype. Clin Pharmacol Ther 45:348–355, 1989

Borga O, Azarnoff DL, Forshell GP, et al: Plasma protein binding of tricyclic antidepressants in man. Biochem Pharmacol 18:2135–2143, 1969

Brosen K, Skjelbo E: Fluoxetine and norfluoxetine are potent inhibitors of P450IID6—the source of the sparteine-debrisoquine oxidation polymorphism (letter). Br J Clin Pharmacol 32:136–137, 1991

Brosen K, Zeugin T, Meyer UA: Role of P450IID6, the target of the sparteine-debrisoquine oxidation polymorphism, in the metabolism of imipramine. Clin Pharmacol Ther 49:609–617, 1991

Downs JM, Dahmer SK: Fluoxetine and elevated plasma levels of tricyclic antidepressants (letter). Am J Psychiatry 147:1251, 1990

Downs JM, Downs AD, Rosenthal TL, et al: Increased plasma tricyclic antidepressant concentrations in two patients concurrently treated with fluoxetine. J Clin Psychiatry 50:226–227, 1989

El-Yazigi A, Chaleby K: Steady-state kinetics of doxepin and imipramine in Saudi patients with interethnic comparison. Psychopharmacology 95:63–67, 1988

Escobar JI, Tuason VB: Antidepressant agents—a cross cultural study. Psychopharmacol Bull 16:49–52, 1980

Gaviria M, Gil AA, Javaid JI: Nortriptyline kinetics in Hispanic and Anglo subjects. J Clin Psychopharmacol 6:227–231, 1986

Hamilton M: A rating scale for depression. J Neurol Neurosurg Psychiatry 23:56–62, 1960

Hammer W, Sjoqvist F: Plasma levels of monomethylated tricyclic antidepressants during treatment with imipramine-like compounds. Life Sci 6:1885–1903, 1967

Henry BW, Overall JE, Markette JR: Comparison of major drug therapies for alleviation of anxiety and depression. Diseases of the Nervous System: 32:655–667, 1971

Hu WH, Lee CF, Yang YY, et al: Imipramine plasma levels and clinical response. Bulletin of Chinese Social Neurosciences and Psychiatry 9:40–49, 1983

Islam SI, Idle JR, Smith RL: The polymorphic 4-hydroxylation of debrisoquine in a Saudi Arab population. Xenobiotica 10:819–825, 1980

Kalow W: Race and therapeutic drug response. N Engl J Med 320:588–589, 1989

Kalow W: Interethnic variation of drug metabolism. Trends Pharmacol Sci 12:102–107, 1991

Kinzie JD, Manson S: Five years' experience with Indochinese refugee psychiatric patients. Journal of Operational Psychiatry 14:13–19, 1983

Kinzie JD, Leung P, Boehnlein JK, et al: Antidepressant blood levels in Southeast Asians—clinical and cultural implications. J Nerv Ment Dis 175:480–485, 1987

Kishimoto A, Hollister LE: Nortriptyline kinetics in Japanese and Americans (letter). J Clin Psychopharmacol 4:171–172, 1984

Kleinman A: Culture and patient care: psychiatry among the Chinese. Drug Ther 11:134–140, 1981

Lewis P, Rack PH, Vaddadi KS, et al: Ethnic differences in drug response. Postgrad Med J 56 (suppl 1):46–49, 1980

Lin KM, Poland RE: Pbarmacotherapy of Asian Psychiatric Patients. Psychiatric Annals 19:659–663, 1989

Livingston RL, Zucker DK, Isenberg K, et al: Tricyclic antidepressants and delirium. J Clin Psychiatry 44:173–176, 1983

Marcos LR, Cancro R: Pharmacotherapy of Hispanic depressed patients: clinical observations. Am J Psychotherapy 36:505–512, 1982

Mellstrom B, Bertilsson L, Sawe J, et al: E and Z 10-hydroxylation of nortriptyline: relationship to polymorphic debrisoquine hydroxylation. Clin Pharmacol Ther 30:189–193, 1981

Mellstrom B, Bertilsson L, Lou YC, et al: Amitriptyline metabolism: relationship to polymorphic debrisoquine hydroxylation. Clin Pharmacol Ther 34:516–520, 1983

Nakamura K, Goto F, Ray WA, et al: Interethnic differences in genetic polymorphism of debrisoquine and mephenytoin hydroxylation between Japanese and Caucasian populations. Clin Pharmacol Ther 38:402–408, 1985

Nordin C, Siwers B, Benitez J, et al: Plasma concentrations of nortiriptyline and its 10-hydroxymetabolite in depressed patients—relationship to debrisoquine hydroxylation metabolic ratio. Br J Clin Pharmacol 19:832–835, 1985

Overall JE, Hollister LE, Kimbell I, et al: Extrinsic factors influencing responses to psychotherapeutic drugs. Arch Gen Psychiatry 21:89–94, 1969

Pi EH, Simpson GH, Cooper MA: Pharmacokinetics of desipramine in Caucasian and Asian volunteers. Am J Psychiatry 143:1174–1176, 1986

Pi EH, Tran-Johnson TK, Walker NR, et al: Pharmacokinetics of desipramine in Asian and Caucasian volunteers. Psychopharmacol Bull 25:483–487, 1989

Potter WZ, Bertilsson L, Sjoqvist F: Handbook of Biological Psychiatry, Part VI. Edited by Van Praag HM, Lader MH, Rafuelsen DJ, et al. New York, Marcel Dekker, 1981, p 71

Preskorn SH, Beber JH, Faul JC, et al: Serious adverse effects of combining fluoxetine and tricyclic antidepressants (letter). Am J Psychiatry 147:532, 1990

Raskin A, Crook TH: Antidepressants in Black and White inpatients. Arch Gen Psychiatry 32:643–649, 1975

Rosenblat R, Tang SW: Do Oriental psychiatric patients receive different dosages of psychotropic medication when compared with Occidentals? Can J Psychiatry 32:270–274, 1987

Rosenstein DL, Takeshita J, Nelson JC: Fluoxetine-induced elevation and prolongation of tricyclic levels in overdose. Am J Psychiatry 148:807, 1991

Rudorfer MV, Robins E: Amitriptyline overdose: clinical effects on tricyclic antidepressant plasma levels. J Clin Psychiatry 43:457–460, 1982

Rudorfer MV, Lane EA, Chang WH, et al: Desipramine pharmacokinetics in Chinese and Caucasian volunteers. Br J Clin Pharmacol 17:433–440, 1984

Rudorfer MV, Lane EA, Potter WZ: Interethnic dissociation between debrisoquine and desipramine hydroxylation. J Clin Psychopharmacol 5:89–92, 1985

Schneider L, Pawluczyk S, Dopheide J, et al: Ethnic differences in nortriptyline metabolism (New Research Program and Abstracts, p 206). Paper presented at the annual meeting of the American Psychiatric Association, New Orleans, LA, May 11–16, 1991

Sjoqvist F, Alexanderson B, Asberg M, et al: Pharmacokinetics and biological effects of nortriptyline in man. Acta Pharmacol Toxicol 29 (suppl 3):255–280, 1971

Skjelbo E, Brosen K, Hallas J, Gram LF: The mephenytoin oxidation polymorphism is partially responsible for the N-demethylation of imipramine. Clin Pharmacol Ther 49:18–23, 1991

Spector R, Choudhury AK, Chiang CK, et al: Diphenhydramine in Orientals and Caucasians. Clin Pharmacol Ther 28:229–234, 1980

Spina E, Birgersson C, von Bahr C, et al: Phenotypic consistency in hydroxylation of desmethylimipramine and debrisoquine in healthy subjects and in human liver microsomes. Clin Pharmacol Ther 36:677–682, 1984

Task Force on the Use of Laboratory Tests in Psychiatry: Tricyclic antidepressants—blood level measurements and clinical outcome: an APA Task Force report. Am J Psychiatry 142(2):155–162, 1985

United Nations: 1986 Demographic Yearbook. New York, Department of International Economic and Social Affairs, Statistical Office, United Nations, 1988

von Ammon Cavanaugh S: Drug-drug interactions of fluoxetine with tricyclics. Psychosomatics 31:273–276, 1990

von Bahr C, Birgersson C, Blanck A, et al: Correlation between nortriptyline and debrisoquine hydroxylation in the human liver. Life Sci 33:631–636, 1983

von Bahr C, Birgersson C, Morgan ET, et al: Oxidation of tricyclic antidepressant drugs, debrisoquine and 7-ethoxyresorufin by human liver preparations. Xenobiotica 16:391–400, 1986

Woolhouse NM, Adjepon-Yamoah KK, Mellstrom B, et al: Nortriptyline and debrisoquine hydroxylations in Ghanaian and Swedish subjects. Clin Pharmacol Ther 36:374–378, 1984

World Health Organization Collaborative Study: Dose effects of antidepressant medication in different populations. J Affective Disord S1–S67, 1986

Yamashita I, Asano Y: Tricyclic antidepressants: therapeutic plasma level. Psychopharmacol Bull 15:40–41, 1979

Zhou HH, Koshakji RP, Silberstein DJ, et al: Racial differences in drug response—altered sensitivity to and clearance of propranolol in men of Chinese descent as compared with American Whites. N Engl J Med 320:565–570, 1989

Ziegler VE, Biggs JT: Tricyclic plasma levels—effect of age, race, sex, and smoking. JAMA 238:2167–2169, 1977

Chapter 5

Ethnicity and Differential Responses to Benzodiazepines

Keh-Ming Lin, M.D., M.P.H.,
Russell E. Poland, Ph.D.,
Joseph C. Fleishaker, Ph.D., and J. Paul Phillips

Since the introduction of chlordiazepoxide into medical practice in 1960, benzodiazepines (BZPs) have become among the most frequently prescribed medications (Smith and Wesson 1985). Surveys in the United States indicated that approximately 15% of the general population have used BZPs within a 1-year period. The use of BZPs accounts for two-thirds of all psychotropic drug use (Greenblatt et al. 1975). Similar studies conducted in various countries indicated that the prevalence of BZP use in the community ranged between 10% and 20% (Parry et al. 1973). This popularity not only reflects the large safety margin of BZPs (especially as compared to their predecessors, the barbiturates) but also their efficacy in treating anxiety and related symptoms (Ballenger 1984; Greenblatt et al. 1983; Lesser 1989; Smith and Wesson 1985). At the same time, because of their potential for abuse and misuse (Noyes et al. 1988; Woods et al. 1987, 1988), their effect on motor and perceptual functioning (Ellinwood and Nikaido 1987), and occasionally their propensity to cause severe withdrawal syndromes (Dupont 1986; Noyes et al. 1988; Woods et al. 1987, 1988), the dosing and prescription patterns of these medications have often been the focus of much scrutiny (Dupont 1986; Greenblatt et al. 1975; Lesser 1989).

Supported in part by MH47355 and Research Center on the Psychobiology of Ethnicity MH47193 (Drs. Lin and Poland), National Institute of Mental Health Research Scientist Development Award MH00534 (Dr. Poland), the Upjohn Company, State of California Contract #85-76263 (Drs. Lin and Poland), and by the National Institutes of Health Clinical Research Center Grant RR00425.

Given the enormity of the issues involved, factors that may affect the response to and dose requirement of BZPs evidently should be carefully examined. Ethnicity has been identified by several clinical and survey reports (Kumana et al. 1987; Murphy 1969, 1972; Rosenblat and Tang 1987) as an important factor in determining BZP responses. Based on his extensive cross-cultural experiences, as well as international surveys, Murphy (1969, 1972) first suggested that, compared to Caucasians, Asians may be more sensitive to the effects of various psychotropics, including anxiolytics. This was supported by a survey of the prescription patterns of 21 American and Canadian psychiatrists who regularly treat both Asian and non-Asian patients (Rosenblat and Tang 1987). The results of this study showed that the mean dosages of BZPs received by Asians were about one-half to two-thirds of those prescribed for their Caucasian counterparts (i.e., diazepam: 12 versus 21 mg/day, $P < .001$; chlordiazepoxide: 32 versus 46 mg/day, $P < .01$). Concurrently, Kumana and colleagues (1987) also indicated that Chinese patients living in Hong Kong generally were treated with substantially small amount of BZPs as compared to Caucasian patients.

In the past decade, a small number of studies have utilized pharmacokinetic, pharmacogenetic, and pharmacodynamic research designs to examine ethnic differences in responses to BZPs. In this chapter, we review these findings and their implications. We then discuss their clinical implications and make suggestions for future research.

PHARMACOKINETIC AND PHARMACODYNAMIC STUDIES

Intravenous Diazepam Study Conducted in St. Louis

Ghoneim and colleagues (1981) studied the kinetics and behavioral effects of diazepam in 12 Caucasian and 13 Asian healthy control subjects. Each subject received 0.2 mg/kg of diazepam intravenously, along with a placebo-control administered in a double-blind fashion. Nine blood samples for the measurement of diazepam and desmethyldiazepam concentrations were obtained over a 72-hour period after treatment. Serum protein binding of diazepam was also determined. Tests of the behavioral and psychological effects of diazepam—including serial learning, subjective ratings, tapping speed, arithmetic test, and delayed recall—were administered three times during the first 4 hours posttreatment.

The results showed that the two ethnic groups diverged substantially in their pharmacokinetic but not their pharmacodynamic responses to diazepam. Significantly slower total body clearance, smaller volume of distribution (V_{area}), and higher levels of desmethyldiazepam concentrations were found in the Asian subjects compared to their Caucasian counterparts. These differences could not be explained by factors such as body weight, nativity (immigration) status, or dietary habits, and were most likely secondary to a less active hepatic metabolism of diazepam in Asians. When extrapolated to the steady state, this difference in the rate of metabolism could lead to Asians having (on the average) 40%–50% higher drug concentrations in serum and in tissue.

There was no difference in the proportion of protein binding (98%) between the two ethnic groups, which was comparable to previous reports in Caucasians. The psychological and behavioral effects of diazepam also were similar in intensity and duration in both groups, which were most prominent at 0.5 hour posttreatment and no longer apparent 4 hours after drug administration. Potential problems in the study design might have prevented the detection of ethnic differences in drug effects. The relatively high dosage of intravenous diazepam used in this study (about 13 mg in Asians and 14 mg in Caucasians) may be too sedating to optimally discern ethnic differences in behavioral or psychological responses; also, the assessment points may not have been frequent enough to catch the maximal response time point. In addition, Ghoneim and colleagues (1981) suggested that although ethnic dynamic difference may be negligible after a single dose of diazepam, it may become substantial after chronic dosing because of the accumulation of the metabolites as well as the parent drug.

Oral Diazepam Study Conducted in Hong Kong

Kumana and colleagues (1987) compared diazepam pharmacokinetics in 16 Chinese and 18 Caucasian healthy male volunteer subjects in Hong Kong. Compared with their Caucasian counterparts, the Chinese subjects were younger, lighter in weight, shorter, and leaner, as judged by skin fold thickness (SFT) (1.14 versus 1.44 cm subscapular, $P = .03$) and total body weight to "ideal" body weight ratio (TBW/IBW) (0.93 versus 1.07, $P = .02$). The Chinese subjects also had lower albumin concentrations (46 versus 50 g/L, $P = .0001$). After screening and collection of the pretreatment blood sample, a 10-mg diazepam (Valium) tablet was administered. This was followed by the collection of a total of 10 blood samples in the next 72 hours at predetermined intervals. Serum concentrations of diazepam and desmethyldiazepam were measured by an enzyme-linked immunoassay for the first 6 samples (0–3 hours) and high-performance liquid chromatography (HPLC) for the last 4 samples (3–72 hours).

The researchers found that T_{max} (time needed to achieve maximal drug concentration) was significantly more prolonged in the Chinese subjects. As reflected by similar peak plasma concentration (C_{max}; actual data not reported) between the two groups, there were no apparent differences in predistribution diazepam concentrations between the two groups. In contrast, the Chinese subjects had 14%–61% higher diazepam and desmethyldiazepam concentrations during the postdistribution period (6–72 hours). They also had a significantly larger first order elimination rate constant (k_e), longer elimination half-life ($t_{1/2}$), and smaller apparent V_{area}. However, when two of these variables, k_e and V_{area}, were treated as dependent variables in a multiple regression analysis, it became evident that the ethnic differences could be largely explained by the differences in SFT and TBW/IBW between the two groups. This suggests that ethnic differences in the percentage of body fat may be the main reason for the higher serum concentrations of diazepam and its metabolite(s) in Asians as compared to Caucasians. Because the serum concentrations of both parent drug (diazepam) and its metabolite (desmethyldiazepam) were lower in Caucasians, Kumana and colleagues (1987) suggested that there was no evidence of differences between the two groups in the activities of liver enzymes responsible for the metabolism of diazepam. Further, because Chinese subjects had longer T_{max} yet higher drug concentrations, the efficiency of gastrointestinal absorption also was not likely to be a relevant factor in this regard.

Oral and Intravenous Alprazolam Study Conducted in Los Angeles

Another study examined plasma alprazolam concentrations and acute behavioral effects in healthy male volunteer subjects, 14 of whom were American-born Asian, 14 foreign-born Asian, and 14 Caucasian (Lin et al. 1988). All subjects were nonsmokers and not regular alcohol drinkers. Subjects were admitted to an inpatient research ward on 2 separate days at least 2 weeks apart. After a 12-hour overnight fast, 0.5 mg alprazolam was administered to the subjects either orally in tablet form with 180 ml of water or as a slow intravenous injection. Prior to drug administration, three baseline blood samples were obtained; over the next 36 hours, 14 posttreatment blood samples were obtained. Plasma derived from these samples were stored at –70°C and assayed for alprazolam concentrations by HPLC. These plasma samples also were used for the determination of growth hormone concentrations by radioimmunoassay (Koulu et al. 1979; Syvalahti and Kanto 1975). Sedation was rated by nurses at the time of each blood sampling. The digital symbol substitute test (DSST; Ellinwood and Nikaido 1987; Greenblatt et al. 1989; Hindmarch 1980; Johnson and Chernik 1982), a psychomotor test previously proven sensitive to the effect of BZPs, was also administered at baseline and again at 2, 4, 6, and 24 hours after the administration of the test drug.

Plasma concentration curves for each individual subject were constructed. The area under the plasma concentration curve (AUC) was then calculated. Also calculated were the peak plasma concentration (C_{max}) and time required to reach the peak concentration (T_{max}), as well as total plasma clearance (CL) and V_{area}.

As shown in Table 5–1, when compared to the Caucasian subjects, both Asian groups had higher AUC and C_{max} and smaller CL after both oral and intravenous administration of alprazolam. These differences either reached statistical significance (AUC and CL after oral administration; C_{max} after intravenous administration) or approached significance (C_{max} after oral administration, AUC after intravenous administration). These statistical differences either remained significant or became significant (for the oral-C_{max} and intravenous-AUC) after body surface area was covaried. Although the $t_{1/2}$ after both oral and intravenous administration of alprazolam was substantially longer in both Asian groups as compared to the Caucasians, these differences failed to reach statistical significance.

In contrast to the differences between the Asian and Caucasian subjects, the pharmacokinetic parameters of the two Asian groups were remarkably similar. There was no significant statistical difference between the two groups in any of the parameters examined.

Although the results derived from pharmacodynamic measurements consistently revealed greater pharmacological effects of alprazolam on Asians as compared to Caucasians, only the differences in the mean sedation scores reached statistical significance, with foreign-born Asians experiencing significantly more

Table 5–1. Comparison of mean pharmacokinetic parameters after oral and intravenous alprazolam administration

	Caucasians[a] (*n* = 14)	**American-born Asians**[a] (*n* = 14)	**Foreign-born Asians**[a] (*n* = 14)	**ANOVA**	
				F	*P*
Oral					
AUC	138 ± 42.0	183 ± 43.8	173 ± 45.0	5.42	.01
C_{max}	9.79 ± 1.49	11.1 ± 2.62	11.7 ± 1.89	3.0	.1
CL	3.91 ± 1.04	2.88 ± 0.68	3.05 ± 0.69	5.4	.01
$t_{1/2}$	12.6 ± 4.05	15.9 ± 4.59	15.8 ± 5.24	2.60	.1
T_{max}	44.4 ± 11.6	69.4 ± 6.05	44.4 ± 11.6	1.37	NS
V_{area}	66.2 ± 10.4	62.5 ± 9.24	65.1 ± 8.15	0.47	NS
Intravenous					
AUC	165 ± 39.2	213 ± 63.7	210 ± 68.7	2.97	.1
C_{max}	12.6 ± 2.04	15.2 ± 2.78	14.4 ± 2.8	3.79	.05
CL	3.17 ± 0.66	2.52 ± 0.69	2.65 ± 1.00	2.58	.1
$t_{1/2}$	13.4 ± 3.42	16.0 ± 5.36	17.8 ± 6.80	2.34	NS
T_{max}	10.9 ± 2.6	12.2 ± 4.1	16.6 ± 2.1	0.55	NS
V_{area}	59.2 ± 10.5	54.2 ± 8.9	60.0 ± 10.4	1.64	NS

Note. Units of measurements: AUC = ng x hour/ml; C_{max} = ng/ml; CL = liter/hour; $t_{1/2}$ = hour; T_{max} = minutes; V_{area} = liter.

[a] Values are means ± SD.

sedation compared to both Caucasian and American-born Asian subjects (Table 5–2). Substantial variances characteristic of studies of this nature have been the main reason for these results.

However, methodological problems may have also contributed to this observation. The relatively low doses of alprazolam (0.5 mg) given to the subjects may not have been sufficient for producing dynamic changes conducive to cross-ethnic comparisons. Further, the DSST performance has been demonstrated to be strongly influenced by educational levels and levels of anxiety. The Caucasian subjects in this study had significantly lower baseline DSST scores than their Asian counterparts, raising the possibility of uneven distribution or discrepancy in education or baseline anxiety levels that could, in turn, complicate the posttreatment findings. To deal with these issues, it may be important to explore the use of other possibly more sensitive dynamic measures and also to attempt to ensure that the comparison groups are more comparable.

Table 5–2. Comparison of mean sedation scores, growth hormone concentrations (ng/ml), and DSST change scores after oral and intravenous alprazolam administration

	Caucasians[a] (n = 14)	**American-born Asians**[a] (n = 14)	**Foreign-born Asians**[a] (n = 14)	**ANOVA** F	P
Oral					
Mean sedation	1.39 ± 0.33	1.54 ± 0.35	1.59 ± 0.37	1.31	NS
Max sedation	2.36 ± 0.74	2.50 ± 0.65	2.57 ± 0.76	.32	NS
Mean GH	0.64 ± 0.88	0.99 ± 1.42	0.81 ± 1.80	.21	NS
Max GH	5.08 ± 5.57	6.86 ± 8.61	7.55 ± 8.93	.40	NS
Mean DSST	3.29 ± 7.10	1.30 ± 8.62	0.18 ± 5.74	.66	NS
Max DSST	–2.00 ± 7.89	–3.79 ± 10.24	6.14 ± 6.63	.86	NS
Intravenous					
Mean sedation	1.48 ± 0.24	1.37 ± 0.23	1.67 ± 0.33	4.45	.018
Max sedation	2.50 ± 0.65	2.36 ± 0.74	2.71 ± 0.47	1.13	NS
Mean GH	1.54 ± 3.02	1.63 ± 1.79	1.81 ± 2.65	.04	NS
Max GH	8.83 ± 13.6	9.84 ± 10.7	12.32 ± 15.89	.25	NS
Mean DSST	4.32 ± 7.21	1.66 ± 7.15	1.93 ± 3.60	.78	NS
Max DSST	–0.64 ± 8.0	–3.43 ± 8.3	–2.86 ± 3.74	.61	NS

Note. GH = growth hormone; DSST = digital symbol substitute test.
[a] Values are means ± SD.

A Pharmacokinetic and Pharmacogenetic Study Conducted in Beijing, China

The cytochrome P_{450} isozymes are involved in the metabolism of most BZPs as well as other psychotropics (Bertilsson et al. 1989; Dahl-Puustinen et al. 1989; Mellstrom et al. 1983; Shen and Lin 1990; Skjelbo et al. 1991). Two of these isozymes, whose activities can be determined with probe drugs such as debrisoquine (Steiner et al. 1988) and S-mephenytoin (Wilkinson et al. 1989), have been found to be polymorphic. Poor metabolizers (PMs) of debrisoquine are extremely rare among Asians (less than 1%; Nakamura et al. 1985) but are relatively common among Caucasian populations (6%–10%). In contrast, the rate of PMs of S-mephenytoin is quite high among Chinese and Japanese (15%–23%) as compared to Caucasians (3%–5%; Horai et al. 1989; Kupfer and Preisig 1984; Wedlund et al. 1984).

Bertilsson and colleagues (1989) demonstrated a high correlation between the metabolism of diazepam and the phenotype status of S-mephenytoin in Caucasian subjects. This finding led to the hypothesis that the higher percentage of S-mephenytoin–type enzyme deficiency among Chinese may be mainly responsible for the slower metabolism of diazepam in this ethnic group. This theory, however, was not supported by a recent report by Zhang and colleagues (1990). In this study, diazepam and demethyldiazepam concentrations were measured over 21 days after the administration of 5 mg of diazepam in 16 healthy Chinese volunteers in Beijing. Among these volunteers, eight were extensive metabolizers (EMs) of S-mephenytoin, the other eight PMs. Other than demethyldiazepam concentrations, which were significantly higher in Chinese EM subjects than in Chinese PM subjects for the whole duration of the study, the two phenotype groups showed no significant difference in most of the pharmacokinetic parameters, including the plasma half-life and clearance of diazepam, which were comparable to Caucasian PMs and drastically different from Caucasian EMs (twice as long for the half-life and only half as fast for the clearance).

The study of Bertilsson and colleagues (1989) thus suggests that the S-mephenytoin hydroxylase present in the Chinese EMs was not able to metabolize diazepam; consequently, unlike the

Caucasian subjects, the metabolism of diazepam among the Chinese subjects was independent of the S-mephenytoin hydroxylation phenotype. It also suggests that the higher incidence of PM of S-mephenytoin in Chinese subjects is not the only factor responsible for the interethnic difference in response to diazepam. Other factors could include differences in substrate specificity of the S-mephenytoin hydroxylase, or the activities of other enzyme systems that are also responsible for the metabolism of diazepam.

Related to this puzzling finding is yet another study (Horai et al. 1989) comparing the metabolic rates of metoprolol (used for testing debrisoquine phenotype) and S-mephenytoin between 200 Japanese subjects living in Japan and 98 Chinese subjects living in the People's Republic of China. Confirming earlier reports, both ethnic groups showed extremely low rates for PM phenotype of debrisoquine-type hydroxylation and a greater incidence of PM phenotype of mephenytoin oxidation. However, Chinese EMs metabolized both drugs significantly slower than did Japanese EMs. It is still unclear whether these differences represent differential environmental influences (differential exposures to various enzyme-inducing agents) or are the results of subtler cross-ethnic differences in the distribution of different variants of the enzymes responsible for the metabolism of these drugs.

In contrast to the Hong Kong study (Kumana et al. 1987), Zhang and colleagues (1990) also reported a larger mean V_{area} in Chinese subjects than in Caucasian subjects. This difference reached statistical significance when Chinese EMs were compared with their Caucasian EM counterparts.

Comparison of the Pharmacokinetics of Adinazolam Between African-Americans and Caucasians

Two of us (Fleishaker and Phillips 1989) conducted a study of the pharmacokinetics and pharmacodynamics of adinazolam, a triazolo-benzodiazepine currently being investigated as an anxiolytic and antidepressant, with eight African-American and eight Caucasian control subjects. The analysis of the pharmacokinetic dose-proportionality and pharmacodynamics in the total population has been published and the results have been reanalyzed to assess ethnic differences in kinetics and dynamics. The results showed that African-Americans had increased clearance of adinazolam, which resulted in a lower AUC, lower C_{max}, and longer half-life in African-Americans compared to Caucasians. Concurrently, however, the C_{max} and AUC of N-demethyladinazolam, a metabolite of adinazolam, were significantly higher in African-Americans. Along with these pharmacokinetic findings, African-Americans also manifested a significantly greater drug effect on psychomotor performance. Adinazolam is almost exclusively eliminated by hepatic oxidation to N-demethyladinazolam. Thus, these findings suggest that African-Americans may have a higher metabolic capacity for adinazolam. Because N-demethyladinazolam is cleared directly by renal excretion in addition to hepatic metabolism (approximately 50% of a dose of adinazolam is recovered in the urine as N-demethyladinazolam), increases in oxidative capacity are expected to have a lesser effect on N-demethyladinazolam AUC values. The increased C_{max} and AUC of N-demethyladinazolam in African-Americans may be due to increased first-pass conversion of adinazolam to N-demethyladinazolam. N-demethyladinazolam has been shown to primarily mediate the BZP-like side effects, including effects on psychomotor performance, after adinazolam administration (Fleishaker et al. 1990, 1992). This may be responsible for the larger drug effects on African-Americans despite their higher metabolic capacity for adinazolam.

CONCLUSION AND FUTURE DIRECTIONS

Five studies have compared the pharmacokinetics and pharmacodynamics of BZPs in different ethnic groups. Among these, four studies involved comparisons between Asians and Caucasians and one study compared African-Americans with Caucasians. At present, to our knowledge, no study has been conducted with other major ethnic groups in this country, such as Hispanics and American Indians. The lack of information in this regard is particularly problematic for several major reasons:

1. These populations, along with Asians and African-Americans, are rapidly growing in this country;
2. BZPs are widely used in practically all ethnic groups in this country as well as worldwide; and
3. Many factors, genetic as well as environmental, could lead to significant ethnic differences in response to BZPs.

All four studies involving Asians and Caucasians demonstrated significant kinetic differences between the two ethnic groups. Because they were conducted at different geographical sites (two in North America, one in Hong Kong, and one in the People's Republic of China) and possibly included different Asian subcultural groups (i.e., not all subjects included in the American studies were of Chinese origin), questions could be raised regarding the generalizability of the findings. At the same time, however, the consistency in these reports of a slower metabolism of BZPs in Asians is quite remarkable, suggesting that perhaps genetic factors are more important than environmental considerations in causing such a phenomenon.

Findings from the two American studies also indirectly point to the importance of genetic influences. Although the results of Zhang and colleagues (1990) were compatible with the hypothesis linking ethnic differences in S-mephenytoin phenotype with BZP metabolism, they also indicated additional mechanisms, either genetic or environmental, that are responsible for the slower elimination rate of diazepam in Chinese EMs of mephenytoin phenotype.

In contrast to the other three studies, Kumana and colleagues (1987) suggested that volume of distribution, secondary to ethnic differences in the percentage of fat in the body, was the major factor for differential ethnic responses to diazepam. However, results from the other studies have not consistently supported such an assertion. Perhaps this inconsistency resulted at least partially from sampling biases. Although the Caucasian subjects included in the study of Kumana and colleagues were older and heavier, the other studies recruited Caucasians whose degree of "fatness" was more comparable to their Asian subjects. However, in clinical situations, this factor may be an additional reason that the majority of Caucasian patients require higher doses of BZPs.

Ghoneim and colleagues (1981) reported no difference in protein binding between their Asian and Caucasian subjects. This was confirmed by a study (Zhou et al. 1990) comparing the protein binding of various drugs, including diazepam, between Asians and Caucasians. Zhou and colleagues further reported that, although there were clear-cut differences between Asians and Caucasians in the concentrations of $alpha_1$ acid glycoprotein, as well as in the degree of protein binding of drugs primarily bound to this plasma protein, the two groups did not differ in their plasma albumin concentrations nor in the proportion of protein binding with drugs primarily bound to albumin. Because most BZPs are bound to albumin, it appears reasonable to believe that protein binding does not represent an important factor in causing ethnic differences in BZP responses.

Although two of the studies (Ghoneim et al. 1981; Lin et al. 1988) included pharmacodynamic measurements, the researchers were not able to detect substantial differences in drug effects, despite the existence of significant ethnic pharmacokinetic differences. This is not surprising, because results of studies conducted by other investigators attempting to correlate dynamic with kinetic parameters of BZPs are not always successful (Ellinwood and Nikaido 1987). More precise and sensitive measurements of drug pharmacodynamics will, one hopes, become available in the near future to help quantify the effects of ethnicity on BZP responses.

Lastly, the absence of studies involving measurement of steady-state plasma drug concentrations in patient populations represents another important issue that needs to be addressed in future research. Although single-dose pharmacokinetic and pharmacodynamic parameters do provide useful information and in general are highly predictive of the steady-state drug levels and effects, such inferences ultimately need to be substantiated with studies that direct and systematically assess the kinetics and effects of the BZPs in the clinical settings.

In summary, newer developments in pharmacokinetics, pharmacogenetics, and pharmacodynamics have made it possible for several research groups to demonstrate significant differences in the metabolism of some of the BZPs between Asians and Caucasians. The mechanisms responsible for such differences remain to be determined, and the findings need to be tested in patient populations receiving BZPs on an ongoing basis. Similar research strategies should be applied to studies involving other ethnic populations. Progress in this area of research should prove significant in the clinical care of the rapidly increasing ethnic minority populations, as well as for the majority of the world's population who are of non-Western backgrounds.

REFERENCES

Ballenger JC: Psychopharmacology of the anxiety disorders. Psychiatr Clin North Am 7:757–771, 1984

Bertilsson L, Henthorn TK, Sanz E, et al: Importance of genetic factors in the regulation of diazepam metabolism: relationship to S-mephenytoin, but not debrisoquine, hydroxylation phenotype. Clin Pharmacol Ther 45:348–355, 1989

Dahl-Puustinen ML, Liden A, Alm C, et al: Disposition of perphenazine is related to polymorphic debrisoquine hydroxylation in human beings. Clin Pharmacol Ther 46:78–81, 1989

Dupont RL: Benzodiazepines: The Social Issues. Rockville, MD, Institute for Behavior and Health, 1986

Ellinwood EH, Nikaido AM: Perceptual-neuromotor pharmacodynamics of psychotropic drugs, in Psychopharmacology: The Third Generation of Progress. Edited by Meltzer HY. New York, Raven, 1987, pp 1457–1466

Fleishaker JC, Phillips JP: Adinazolam pharmacokinetics and behavioral effects following administration of 20–60 mg oral doses of its mesylate salt in healthy volunteers. Psychopharmacol 99:34–39, 1989

Fleishaker JC, Friedman H, Pollock SR, et al: Clinical pharmacology of adinazolam and N-desmethyladinazolam mesylate after single oral doses of each compound in healthy volunteers. Clin Pharmacol Ther (reprint)48:652–664, 1990

Fleishaker JC, Smith TC, Friedman HL, et al: Separation of the pharmacokinetic/pharmacodynamic properties of oral and iv adinazolam mesylate and N-desmethyladinazolam mesylate in healthy volunteers. Drug Investigations 4:155–165, 1992

Ghoneim MM, Korttila K, Chiang CK, et al: Diazepam effects and kinetics in Caucasians and Orientals. Clin Pharmacol Ther 29:749–756, 1981

Greenblatt DJ, Shader RI, Koch-Weser J: Psychotropic drug use in the Boston area: a report from the Boston Collaborative Drug Surveillance Program. Arch Gen Psychiatry 32:518–521, 1975

Greenblatt DJ, Shader RI, Abernathy DR: Drug therapy: current status of the benzodiazepines. N Engl J Med 309:354–358, 410–416, 1983
Greenblatt DJ, Harmatz JS, Engelhardt N, et al: Pharmacokinetic determinants of dynamic differences among three benzodiazepine hypnotics. Arch Gen Psychiatry 46:326–330, 1989
Hindmarch I: Psychomotor function and psychoactive drugs. Br J Clin Pharmacol 10:189–209, 1980
Horai Y, Nakano M, Ishizaki T, et al: Metoprolol and mephenytoin oxidation polymorphisms in Far Eastern Oriental subjects: Japanese versus mainland Chinese. Clin Pharmacol Ther 46:198–207, 1989
Johnson LC, Chernik DA: Sedative-hypnotics and human performance. Psychopharmacology 76:101–113, 1982
Koulu M, Lammintausta R, Kangas L, et al: The effect of methysergide, pimozide, and sodium valproate on the diazepam-stimulated growth hormone secretion in man. J Clin Endocrinol Metab 48:119–122, 1979
Kumana CR, Lauder IJ, Chan M, et al: Differences in diazepam pharmacokinetics in Chinese and White Caucasians—relation to body lipid stores. Eur J Clin Pharmacol 32:211–215, 1987
Kupfer A, Preisig R: Pharmacogenetics of mephenytoin: a new drug hydroxylation polymorphism in man. Eur J Clin Pharmacol 26:753–759, 1984
Lesser IM: Legal issues and the benzodiazepines. American Journal of Forensic Psychiatry 10:5–13, 1989
Lin KM, Lau JK, Smith R, et al: Comparison of alprazolam plasma levels and behavioral effects in normal Asian and Caucasian male volunteers. Psychopharmacology (Berlin) 96:365–369, 1988
Mellstrom B, Bertilsson L, Lou YC, et al: Amitriptyline metabolism: relationship to polymorphic debrisoquine hydroxylation. Clin Pharmacol Ther 34:516–520, 1983
Murphy HBM: Ethnic variations in drug responses. Transcultural Psychiatric Research Review 6:6–23, 1969
Murphy HBM: Psychopharmacologie et Variations Ethnoculturelles. Confrontation Psychiatrique 9:163–185. Abstracted in English (1974) in Transcultural Psychiatric Research Review 11:28–31, 1972
Nakamura K, Goto F, Ray WA, et al: Interethnic differences in genetic polymorphism of debrisoquine and mephenytoin hydroxylation between Japanese and Caucasian populations. Clin Pharmacol Ther 38:402–408, 1985
Noyes R, Garvery MJ, Cook BL, et al: Benzodiazepine withdrawal: a review of the evidence. J Clin Psychiatry 49:382–389, 1988
Parry HJ, Balter MB, Mellinger GD, et al: National patterns of psychotherapeutic drug use. Arch Gen Psychiatry 28:769–783, 1973

Rosenblat R, Tang SW: Do Oriental psychiatric patients receive different dosages of psychotropic medication when compared with Occidentals? Can J Psychiatry 32:270–274, 1987

Shen WW, Lin KM: Cytochrome P-450 monooxygenases and interactions of psychotropic drugs. Int J Psychiatry Med 21:21–30, 1990

Skjelbo E, Brosen K, Hallas J, et al: The mephenytoin oxidation polymorphism is partially responsible for the N-demethylation of imipramine. Clin Pharmacol Ther 49:18–23, 1991

Smith DE, Wesson DR (eds): The Benzodiazepines: Current Standards for Medical Practice. Lancaster, England, MTP Press Ltd, 1985

Steiner E, Bertilsson L, Sawe J, et al: Polymorphic debrisoquine hydroxylation in 757 Swedish subjects. Clin Pharmacol Ther 44:431–435, 1988

Syvalahti E, Kanto J: Serum growth hormone, serum immunoreactive insulin and blood glucose response to oral and intravenous diazepam in man. Int J Clin Pharmacol 12:74, 1975

Wedlund PJ, Aslanian WS, McAllister CB, et al: Mephenytoin hydroxylation deficiency in Caucasians: frequency of a new oxidative drug metabolism polymorphism. Clin Pharmacol Ther 36:773–780, 1984

Wilkinson GR, Guengerich FP, Branch RA: Genetic polymorphism of S-mephenytoin hydroxylation. Pharmacol Ther 43:53–76, 1989

Woods JH, Katz JL, Winger GD: Abuse liability of benzodiazepines. Pharmacol Rev 39:251–413, 1987

Woods JH, Katz JL, Winger G: Use and abuse of benzodiazepines: issues relevant to prescribing. JAMA 260:3476–3480, 1988

Zhang Y, Reviriego J, Lou Y, et al: Diazepam metabolism in native Chinese poor and extensive hydroxylators of S-mephenytoin: interethnic differences in comparison with white subjects. Clin Pharmacol Ther 48:496–502, 1990

Zhou HH, Adedoyin A, Wilkinson GR: Differences in plasma binding of drugs between Caucasians and Chinese subjects. Clin Pharmacol Ther 48:10–17, 1990

Chapter 6

Interethnic Variation in Response to Lithium Therapy Among African-American and Asian-American Populations

Tony L. Strickland, Ph.D., William Lawson, M.D., Ph.D., Keh-Ming Lin, M.D., M.P.H., and Paul Fu, Ph.D.

Recent research developments in psychopharmacology reveal significant interethnic variation in response to an array of psychotropic agents (Lin et al. 1990; Wood and Zhou 1991). Although, in comparison, far more investigations of differential interethnic pharmacologic response have been demonstrated with nonpsychoactive than psychoactive medications (Kalow et al. 1986), important differences between groups in response to psychotropics are emerging nonetheless. It has been adequately documented that the pharmacogenetic and pharmacokinetic properties of psychotropics and nonpsychotropics share similar metabolic pathways (Kalow 1982; Lin et al. 1986). As a result, it is not surprising that differences also have been reported to occur with psychoactive compounds, though not in a systematic manner across all types of psychotropics.

However, one area of psychopharmacology research where ethnic differences in responses have been fairly consistently demonstrated is with lithium. This literature suggests significant ethnic variation among Asian, African-American, and Caucasian groups. For example, African-Americans have less efficient cell membrane lithium-sodium countertransport ability and rela-

Supported in part by the Research Center on the Psychobiology of Ethnicity MH47193 (Drs. Strickland and Lin) and NHLBI MSFDA Award HL01988-03 (Dr. Strickland).

tively higher red blood count (RBC)-to-plasma lithium ratios compared to Caucasians. In this chapter, we review the extant literature on interethnic variations in response to lithium in African-American and Asian populations when compared to Caucasian samples. We conclude with our impressions as to how those findings may relate to clinical management of these populations.

CLINICAL INDICATIONS FOR LITHIUM THERAPY

Lithium salts have been widely used to treat psychiatric disorders since their clinical efficacy for mania was shown by John Cade (1949). Numerous studies have shown that lithium carbonate is effective in the treatment of manic episodes and superior to antipsychotics in treating acute mania (Janicak et al. 1992). Moreover, lithium is the treatment of choice for the prophylaxis of bipolar affective disorder (Janicak and Boshes 1987).

Case studies and open clinical trials (but few double-blind controlled studies) have also shown lithium to be useful in a variety of disorders that can be characterized as cyclical or intermittent, including intermittent explosive disorder and cycloid psychosis (Conn and Lion 1984). Lithium seems to reduce violent or impulsive behavior irrespective of etiology (i.e., in personality disorder or organic brain disorder; Janicak and Boshes 1987).

Lithium is also widely used as an adjunctive medication. It may improve the responsiveness of schizophrenic patients concurrently on neuroleptics (Delva and Letamendia 1982). Finally, some patients who have been refractory to antidepressant treatment will improve when given both lithium and the antidepressant (Price et al. 1986).

In summary, it is well established that lithium is effective in the treatment of bipolar disorder. Usually a good therapeutic response is achieved between 0.7 and 1.3 mEq/L, with the upper limit heavily dependent on toxicity. However, there exists significant interethnic variation in relation to plasma levels and subsequent therapeutic response.

PHARMACOKINETIC VARIATION TO LITHIUM IN AFRICAN-AMERICAN POPULATIONS

A number of studies have suggested that the lithium variation in African-Americans is related to a less efficient RBC lithium-sodium countertransport pathway in this group (Trevisan et al. 1984). This observation is significant in that the issue of neurotoxicity has remained a major concern in the management of patients being treated with lithium. These studies have sought a better understanding of the kinetics and clinical effects in mood disorders. However, until recently, comparatively fewer research efforts have focused on interethnic variation in the kinetics of lithium as a potentially significant mediator in therapeutic response and outcome.

As previously noted, there have been varying reports in the literature suggesting that the intra-RBC lithium levels and RBC/serum lithium ratios differ between blacks and Caucasians (Chang et al. 1984; Okpaku et al. 1980; Ostrow et al. 1986).

In a well-controlled investigation, Okpaku and colleagues (1980) studied African-American and Caucasian control subjects who were free of all medications for at least 2 weeks and had no personal or familial history of psychiatric disorders, including alcohol and drug abuse. Blood samples were drawn from each subject, and the RBCs were separated and loaded with lithium. Spectrophotometry was used to measure RBC lithium and sodium at 0 and 25 hours. The RBC lithium concentration levels were virtually identical between African-Americans and Caucasians immediately after loading. However, after 25 hours, the lithium levels were significantly higher in the RBCs of African-American subjects, indicating that the lithium efflux rate was lower, and the lithium RBC/plasma ratio was higher in African-American than in Caucasian subjects. A study by Chang and colleagues (1984) with 30 Caucasian and 13 African-American patients receiving steady-state lithium also confirmed this observation. Further, an in vivo study by Fu and colleagues (1991) compared lithium ratio in 28 Caucasian, 11 African-American, and 8 Asian bipolar patients who had no history of drug abuse and were responsive to lithium treatment. The lithium ratio was again found significantly higher in African-Americans than in

Caucasians and Asians. There were no statistically significant differences in the lithium ratio between Caucasians and Asians. This preliminary finding further supports previous reports.

Intra-RBC lithium concentrations are believed to correspond to intraneuronal lithium concentrations (Elizur et al. 1972). The existence of a higher RBC/plasma lithium ratio in African-Americans suggests that in order to achieve similar intracellular lithium concentrations, the serum (extracellular) lithium concentrations and hence the dosage of lithium for African-American patients may need to be lower. Because studies have suggested that intracellular lithium concentrations may be correlated with the incidence of toxic side effects of lithium (Hewick and Murray 1976; Ostrow et al. 1986; Zakowska-Dabrowska and Rybakowski 1973), a consistent demonstration of interethnic differences in RBC/plasma ratios may have profound clinical implications.

In addition to an ethnic difference in lithium ratio, Chang and colleagues (1984) also demonstrated a statistically significantly longer lithium half-life in African-American subjects (20.9 hours) as compared to Caucasian (15.9 hours) and Chinese (14.1 hours) subjects. However, the estimation of the half-life in this study was based only on 2 time-points (12 and 25 hours after dosing) and thus may be subject to a greater likelihood of error. In another study, Shelley (1987) compared the pharmacokinetics of lithium between 10 Afro-Caribbean and 11 Caucasian subjects. Although Afro-Caribbean subjects had higher lithium concentration and slower elimination, these differences did not reach statistical significance.

To summarize, the research on African-Americans and Afro-Caribbeans regarding lithium pharmacokinetics indicates that they have less efficient cell membrane sodium-lithium countertransport and higher RBC/plasma lithium ratios. Additionally, although there was some evidence suggesting that lithium may be excreted more slowly in African-Americans and Afro-Caribbeans, this has not been consistently confirmed. Although the difference in lithium ratio suggests that African-Americans and Afro-Caribbeans may need less lithium than is currently administered to achieve control over symptomatology, this hypothesis remains to be tested with more vigorously designed prospective clinical studies.

PHARMACOKINETIC VARIATION TO LITHIUM IN ASIAN POPULATIONS

For more than 20 years, lithium has been widely used in various Asian countries for the treatment of bipolar disorder. Although the efficacy of the medicine in treatment of Asians appears to be similar to that reported for non-Asians in Western settings (Lin et al. 1986, 1990), the dosage and therapeutic concentrations of lithium required for patients have been consistently found to be substantially lower than those usually prescribed in Europe, the United States, and Canada. This was first described by Takahashi (1979) and Okuma (1981), who found that patients in Japan with manic-depressive disorder responded to lower doses of lithium, with correspondingly lower therapeutic blood levels of 0.4–0.8 mEq/L.

Subsequently, Yang (1985) studied 101 Taiwanese bipolar patients treated over a 2-year period with clinically determined doses of lithium. He found that 62 of the patients with less variation of lithium levels (less than 0.2 mEq/L) responded significantly better to the treatment than those with a variation higher than 0.2 mEq/L. When analysis was limited to those 62 patients with stable lithium levels, Yang found that the lithium level of the majority of patients who were good responders ranged between 0.5 and 0.79 mEq/L. In two studies conducted separately in Shanghai, China, and in Taipei, Taiwan, Chang and colleagues (1984, 1985) reported remarkably similar therapeutic lithium concentrations for these two Chinese groups residing in drastically divergent socioeconomic environments (0.73 and 0.71 mEq/L, respectively). These were significantly lower than the mean level of 0.98 mEq/L for the matched Caucasian-American patients, as well as the 0.8 to 1.2 mEq/L therapeutic levels generally reported in Europe, the United States, and Canada (Jefferson et al. 1987).

In contrast to the substantial differences in the therapeutic dose range and serum concentrations of lithium between Asians and Caucasians, there appears to be no pharmacokinetic differences between the two ethnic groups. Honda and Suzuki (1979) and Chang and colleagues (1984) reported, respectively, that steady-state pharmacokinetics of lithium in Japanese in Japan and Chinese in Shanghai were similar to data reported for subjects in Western countries. Chang and colleagues (1985) further conducted a single-dose kinetics study of lithium between 22 Taiwanese Chinese and 30 Caucasian bipolar patients. All patients went through washout for at least 1 week prior to the study. Serial serum lithium concentrations were then determined for up to 31 hours after a single 900-mg dose of lithium carbonate. The researchers found that the two ethnic groups did not differ in terms of all the kinetic parameters calculated. Chang and colleagues also reported no differences in RBC/plasma lithium ratio between Chinese and Caucasian subjects.

Together, these studies suggested that although Asians and Caucasians do not differ in lithium kinetics, they diverge in dosage requirement and therapeutic concentrations because of pharmacodynamic reasons. However, this interpretation remains a hypothesis requiring further testing for at least two important reasons: 1) the lack of a fixed-dose design in the clinical studies cited previously, and the possible confounding influence of concomitant use of other medications such as neuroleptics and tricyclic antidepressants; and 2) reports by several experts in Europe (Coppen et al. 1983; Hullin 1980) suggesting that lithium concentrations in the range comparable to those reported in Asian countries may be sufficient for the prophylaxis of manic episodes for Western patients as well. However, in a random assignment double-blind prospective study in the United States (ethnicity of patients not specified) comparing standard (0.8 to 1.0 mmol/L) versus low-range (0.4–0.6 mmol/L) serum lithium levels, Keller and colleagues (1992) found that the standard level group was significantly less likely to experience a relapse of bipolar disorder.

CULTURAL FACTORS IN THE PHARMACOTHERAPY OF LITHIUM

Clinical Treatment Issues in Ethnic Minorities

In treating racial and ethnic minorities, one of the first considerations should be to determine whether lithium treatment is indeed indicated. On the surface, this appears to be a mundane issue.

However, the current literature suggests that lithium may be underprescribed among certain racial and ethnic minorities. By way of illustration, antipsychotics may be overprescribed, because African-Americans and Hispanics with bipolar affective disorder are at a greater risk of receiving a misdiagnosis of schizophrenia (Jones and Gary 1986; Lawson 1986). Mukhersee and colleagues (1981) compared previous diagnoses of African-American, Hispanic, and Caucasian bipolar patients whose diagnosis had been established with the use of DSM-III (American Psychiatric Association 1980) criteria. The researchers found that significantly more African-American and Hispanic patients had received a diagnosis of schizophrenia in the past. Misdiagnosis had significant treatment implications. Bell and Mehta (Bell 1986; Bell and Mehta 1980a, 1980b) reported that manic African-American patients who were misdiagnosed as schizophrenic were far more likely to receive antipsychotics in lieu of lithium therapy. Because some controlled studies show lithium to be more effective than antipsychotics in the treatment of acute mania (Janicak et al. 1992), not surprisingly, these patients showed a poorer treatment response and outcome. In addition to suboptimal treatment, patients treated with antipsychotics also run an increased risk for developing extrapyramidal side effects, including the persisting and sometimes irreversible movement disorder, tardive dyskinesia.

The issue of diagnostic misclassification is not specific to the Caucasian clinician–black patient dyad. In a study of young African-American and Caucasian clinicians' impressions of African-American and Caucasian patients matched for diagnoses, Strickland and colleagues (1988) found that African-American patients were not rated differently on severity of psychopathology but rather on factors closely related to the impression formation process. African-Americans were viewed as less verbally skilled and less "appropriate for therapy" than their Caucasian counterparts. Contrary to expectations, Caucasian clinicians tended to underrate the pathology of African-American patients. On the other hand, African-American clinicians tended to overrate the pathology of Caucasian patients and evince mixed judgments of African-American patients. Regardless, the potentially dire consequence of such diagnostic impressions would be to ignore actual psychopathology in African-Americans and potentially withhold treatment when it is needed.

In view of the persistent problem of misdiagnosis, the clinician should give careful attention to minority patients who are diagnosed as having schizophrenia or other psychosis with a history of poor antipsychotic response, prominent affective features, periodic episodes, or a poorly defined history of schizophreniform symptoms. Such patients deserve a careful, systematic evaluation, preferably with the use of a structured interview instrument such as the Structured Clinical Interview for DSM-III-R (American Psychiatric Association 1987; Spitzer et al. 1990). When in doubt, lithium may be added to the antipsychotic as a therapeutic trial. If the history is highly suggestive of a bipolar disorder, a trial of lithium alone should be considered.

The criminal justice system and various psychosocial interventions outside of the traditional mental health system are often used to address individuals with antisocial behavior and conduct disturbances in the minority community. However, Bell (1986) has made a compelling argument for an organic etiology in some of these cases. He and other researchers have noted that African-Americans are at increased risk for head injury and coma (Bell 1986; Lewis et al. 1986), which may contribute to impulsivity and violent behavior in some cases. A lithium trial should be considered in some of these cases because of lithium's demonstrated effects on impulsive and explosive behavior in individuals with organic brain injury. Because African-Americans and Hispanics are more likely than Caucasians from the same referral source to receive a diagnosis of antisocial personality or to be sent to the criminal justice system than the mental health system (Lewis et al. 1989), lithium should be considered even for a population in corrections. In addition, a number of studies (Cohen and Niska 1980; Krauthammer and Klerman 1978; Robinson et al. 1988) have also indicated that brain injury increases the risk of mania, further strengthening the rationale of a trial of lithium in some of these patients. This is not to say that social factors are unimportant or that there is no role for individual responsibility. Rather, head injury or other organic etiology may interact with social factors, and agents such as lithium may positively affect the response to psychosocial intervention.

Therapeutic Monitoring

Lithium requires appropriate plasma levels to be efficacious. Moreover, it has a narrow therapeutic index, and regular plasma monitoring is therefore necessary to prevent toxicity. Also, lithium is commonly used chronically to prevent relapse. Monitoring is one way to ensure compliance.

To date, there have been no reports of black-Caucasian or Asian-Caucasian differences in clinical response to lithium. Nevertheless, African-Americans show a significantly longer plasma lithium half-life and a higher erythrocyte-to-plasma ratio of lithium than do Caucasians (Chang et al. 1984) or Asians. The clinical significance of this finding is not known. However, the longer plasma half-life may influence the oral dose. With lithium's narrow therapeutic index, care should be taken in prescribing to avoid toxicity. Even mild toxicity may lead to poor compliance. A careful check of therapeutic levels and a switch in the dosage regimen may be necessary.

In order to effectively prevent relapse, lithium must be taken on a regular basis to maintain therapeutic blood levels. Consequently, compliance is extremely important. However, because prophylaxis essentially involves chronic medication use in the absence of symptoms, issues of compliance frequently arise. The problem of treatment compliance is generally substantial and is often further aggravated in cross-ethnic therapeutic situations (Thomas and Sillen 1972; see also Chapter 3). There is evidence that poor compliance may contribute to the increased likelihood of African-American males receiving depot (long-lasting weekly or monthly injections) rather than daily oral medication (Price et al. 1985). Any clinician should be particularly cognizant of the therapeutic relationship as a means of enhancing compliance when working with culturally dissimilar patients (Strickland et al. 1988).

The erythrocyte/plasma ratio has been associated with neuroleptic-lithium–induced toxicity (Pandy et al. 1979), a relatively rare phenomenon in which toxicity is seen with normally therapeutic plasma levels of lithium (Spring and Frankel 1981; Tupin and Schuller 1978). Consequently, clinicians should take care to identify early signs of toxicity, either by symptom or physical history, even when blood levels are not excessive. Asians and Hispanics reportedly require lower lithium dosages (Pandy et al. 1979), but a pharmacokinetic basis for these differences has not been demonstrated. Overall, these findings suggest that dosing should be related to careful monitoring of lithium plasma levels. Careful evaluation for side effects should be done even when plasma levels are within therapeutic levels.

Nearly 25% of African-Americans develop hypertension (Epstein 1967). Some treatments of hypertension can significantly affect lithium plasma levels and the risk for toxicity. Salt restriction can reduce lithium excretion and increase lithium levels to toxicity on a fixed dose (Gibson and Gibbons 1982). Lithium should be avoided, or cautiously managed and monitored, when a severely restrictive high-salt diet is necessary. Thiazide diuretics are less expensive and believed to be superior to other antihypertensive medication for African-Americans, and they are often prescribed in the treatment of hypertension (Freis et al. 1988). Thiazide diuretics also reduce lithium elimination, leading to an elevation of plasma levels (Gibson and Gibbons 1982). When lithium and thiazide diuretics are taken together, the lithium levels should be carefully monitored.

Lithium is eliminated primarily through the kidneys, and long-term use leads to polyuria and secretion of dilute urine. Morphological renal changes may be seen in up to 20% of lithium users but are usually benign (Vestergoard et al. 1982). These changes generally consist of an impairment in water reabsorption. Thus far, no studies have shown a link between lithium and severe renal disease (Gibson and Gibbons 1982). However, these studies seldom identify ethnicity. More care probably should be taken with African-American patients. As noted previously, one-quarter of African-Americans have hypertension, and African-Americans have an increased risk for renal disease, which may be a consequence of the increased prevalence of hypertension (Gibson and Gibbons 1982). Although no research thus far has evaluated relative risk for kidney failure of African-Americans on lithium, it would be prudent for the clinician treating African-American patients to be especially diligent in regularly monitoring the patients' renal function, especially in individuals with hypertension.

In general, the literature suggests that minority patients, particularly African-Americans, should have dosing done less aggressively and have a more careful medical follow-up until these issues are resolved by more research.

Future Directions

Overall, a number of questions need further investigation. First, the pharmacokinetics and pharmacodynamics of lithium in African-Americans and Asian-Americans need further research. We noted previously that African-Americans are less likely to be in pharmacology studies or studies of biological markers in psychiatry. Additional research in general is needed to examine the role of lithium in nonaffective disorders, because it may be a better tolerated alternative to long-term use of antipsychotics. In view of the increased prevalence and perhaps different etiological basis for hypertension in African-Americans, more research is needed on the renal effects of lithium in this population. Finally, more research is needed in health policy research to determine if African-Americans have the necessary access to lithium treatment and to identify barriers that may prevent this access.

SUMMARY AND CONCLUSIONS

Recent advances in psychopharmacology have facilitated some interesting and provocative interethnic comparisons of pharmacogenetic, pharmacokinetic, and pharmacodynamic differences between patient groups. We reviewed the extant psychopharmacology literature demonstrating variation to lithium between Asians and blacks when compared with Caucasians. Although there exist some methodological and other research design concerns that make more definitive impressions premature, there is nonetheless an emerging body of data that identifies significant differential patterns of kinetic and dynamic responsivity to lithium.

Interethnic differences in response to lithium are in their nascency relative to empirical evaluation. Nonetheless, the findings demonstrated thus far with lithium as well as other psychotropic medications in Asians and African-Americans would suggest that significant differences may be overlooked.

One area where well-controlled studies of pharmacokinetic differences have been fairly consistently demonstrated is with lithium. This literature suggests that blacks have less efficient cell membrane lithium-sodium countertransport ability and higher RBC/plasma lithium ratios. Differences in the cellular lithium efflux rate in blacks are highly suggestive, though they need to be confirmed by more extensive studies.

Much work is needed to clearly delineate these important interethnic differences. Future psychopharmacology studies should control for the influences of socioecological factors such as patient nutritional status, diet, smoking behavior, and alcohol and illicit drug use, all of which may individually or collectively affect the pharmacokinetics and/or pharmacogenetics of psychotropics. These factors are important in the study of any interethnic pharmacokinetic comparison, and they are particularly important in the study of black patients because of strong environmental interactions coupled with the extensive intragroup gene pool variation. Accounting for such factors will undoubtedly have direct ramifications for studying interethnic psychopharmacologic differences in blacks and any other ethnic or racial group.

REFERENCES

American Psychiatric Association: Diagnostic and Statistical Manual of Mental Disorders, 3rd Edition. Washington, DC, American Psychiatric Association, 1980

American Psychiatric Association: Diagnostic and Statistical Manual of Mental Disorders, 3rd Edition, Revised. Washington, DC, American Psychiatric Association, 1987

Bell CC: Coma and the etiology of violence, part 1. J Natl Med Assoc 78:1167–1176, 1986

Bell CC, Mehta H: The misdiagnosis of Black patients with manic depressive illness. J Natl Med Assoc 72:141–145, 1980a

Bell CC, Mehta H: Misdiagnoses of Black patients with manic depressive illness: second in the series. J Natl Med Assoc 73:101–107, 1980b

Cade JF: Lithium salts in the treatment of psychotic excitement. Med J Aust 36:349–352, 1949

Chang SS, Pandy GN, Davis JM, et al: Racial differences in plasma and RBC lithium levels. Paper presented at the annual meeting of the American Psychiatric Association, Continuing Medical Education Syllabus and Scientific Proceedings, 1984, pp 239–240

Chang SS, Pandy GN, Yang YY, et al: Lithium pharmacokinetics: interracial comparison. Paper presented at the 138th Annual Meeting of the American Psychiatric Association, Dallas, Texas, May 19–24, 1985

Cohen MR, Niska RW: Localized right cerebral hemisphere dysfunction and recurrent mania. Am J Psychiatry 137:847–848, 1980

Conn L, Lion JR: Psychopharmacology of violence. Psychiatr Clin North Am 7:879–886, 1984

Coppen A, Abou-Saleh M, Miller P, et al: Decreasing lithium dosage reduces morbidity and side-effects during prophylaxis. J Affective Disord 5:353–362, 1983

Delva N, Letamendia F: Lithium treatment in schizophrenic and schizoaffective disorders. Br J Psychiatry 141:387–400, 1982

Elizur A, Shopsin B, Gershon S, et al: Intra: extracellular lithium ratios and clinical course in affective states. Clin Pharmacol Ther 13:947–952, 1972

Epstein FH: The epidemiology of high blood pressure: geographical distributions and etiological factors, in The Epidemiology of Hypertension. Edited by Stamler J, Stamler R, Pullman T. New York, Grune & Stratton, 1967, pp 155–166

Freis ED, Reda DJ, Materson BJ: Volume (weight) loss and blood pressure response followed by thiazide diuretics. Hypertension 12:244–250, 1988

Fu P, Strickland T, Lin KM, et al: RBC/plasma lithium ratio differences in ethnicity. Presented at the Second Annual International Meeting, Pacific Rim Association for Clinical Pharmacogenetics, Los Angeles, CA, October 23–24, 1991

Gibson GS, Gibbons A: Hypertension among Blacks. Hypertension 4:3–51, 1982

Hewick DS, Murray N: Red blood cell levels and lithium toxicity. Lancet 2:473, 1976

Honda Y, Suzuki T: Transcultural pharmacokinetic study on Li concentration in plasma and saliva. Psychopharmacol Bull 15:37–39, 1979

Hullin RP: Minimum serum lithium levels for effective prophylaxis, in Handbook of Lithium Therapy. Edited by Johnson FN. Lancaster, England, MTP Press Ltd, 1980, pp 243–247

Janicak PG, Boshes RA: Advances in the advances of mania and other acute psychotic disorders. Psychiatric Annals 17:145–149, 1987

Janicak PG, Newman RH, Davis JM: Advances in the treatment of mania and related disorders; a reappraisal. Psychiatric Annals 22:92–103, 1992

Jefferson JW, Greist JH, Ackerman DL, et al (eds): Lithium Encyclopedia for Clinical Practice, 2nd Edition. Washington, DC, American Psychiatric Press, 1987

Jones BE, Gary BA: Problems in diagnosing schizophrenia and affective disorders among Blacks. Hosp Community Psychiatry 37:61–65, 1986

Kalow W: Ethnic differences in drug metabolism. Clin Pharmacokinet 7:373–400, 1982

Kalow W, Goedde HW, Agarwal DP (eds): Ethnic Differences in Reactions to Drugs and Xenobiotics: Proceedings of a Meeting Held in Titisee, Black Forest, Federal Republic of Germany, October 3–6, 1985. New York, Alan R Liss, 1986

Keller MB, Lavori PW, Kane JM, et al: Subsyndromal symptoms in bipolar disorder: a comparison of standard and low serum levels of lithium. Arch Gen Psychiatry 49:371–376, 1992

Krauthammer C, Klerman GL: Secondary mania: manic syndromes associated with antecedent physical illness or drugs. Arch Gen Psychiatry 35:1333–1339, 1978

Lawson WB: Racial and ethnic factors in psychiatric research. Hosp Community Psychiatry 37:50–54, 1986

Lewis DO, Pincus JH, Feldman M, et al: Psychiatry neurological and psychoeducational characteristics of 15 death row inmates in the United States. Am J Psychiatry 143:838–845, 1986

Lewis DO, Shanok SS, Cohen RJ, et al: Race bias in the diagnosis and disposition of violent adolescents, Am J Psychiatry 137:1216–1221, 1989

Lin KM, Poland RE, Lesser IM: Ethnicity and psychopharmacology. Cult Med Psychiatry 10:151–165, 1986

Lin KM, Poland RE, Chien CP: Ethnicity and psychopharmacology: recent findings and future research directions, in Family, Culture and Psychobiology. Edited by Sorrel E. New York, Legas, 1990, pp 111–131

Mukhersee S, Shukla S, Woodle J: Misdiagnosis of Schizophrenia in bipolar patients: a multi-ethnic comparison. Am J Psychiatry 138:654–657, 1981

Okpaku S, Fraxer A, Mendels J: A pilot study of racial differences in erythrocyte lithium transport. Am J Psychiatry 137:120–121, 1980

Okuma T: Differential sensitivity to the effects of psychotropic drugs: psychotics vs. normals; Asians vs. Western populations. Folia Psychiatrica et Neurologica Japonica 35:79–81, 1981

Ostrow DG, Dorus W, Okonek A, et al: The effect of alcoholism on membrane lithium transport. J Clin Psychiatry 47:350–353, 1986
Pandy GN, Goel I, Davis JM: Effects of neuroleptic drugs on Lithium uptake by the human erythrocyte. Clin Pharmacol Ther 26:96–102, 1979
Price LH, Charney DS, Heninger DR: Variability of response to Lithium augmentation in refractory depression. Am J Psychiatry 143:1387–1392, 1986
Price N, Glazer W, Morgenstern H: Demographic predictors of the use of injectable versus oral antipsychotic medications in outpatients. Am J Psychiatry 142:1491–1492, 1985
Robinson RG, Boston JD, Starkstein SE, et al: Comparison of mania and depression after brain injury: causal factors. Am J Psychiatry 145:172–178, 1988
Shelley RK: Are there ethnic differences in lithium pharmacokinetics and side-effects? Int Clin Psychopharmacol 2:337–342, 1987
Spitzer RL, Williams JBW, Gibbon M, et al: Structured Clinical Interview for DSM-III-R. Washington, DC, American Psychiatric Press, 1990
Spring G, Frankel M: New data on lithium and haloperidol incompatibility. Am J Psychiatry 138:818–821, 1981
Strickland TL, Jenkins JO, Myers HF, et al: Diagnostic judgments as a function of client and therapist race. Journal of Psychopathology and Behavioral Assessment 10:141–151, 1988
Takahashi R: Lithium treatment in affective disorders: therapeutic plasma level. Psychopharmacol Bull 15:32–35, 1979
Thomas A, Sillen S: Racism and Psychiatry. New York, Brunner/Mazel, 1972
Trevisan M, Ostrow D, Cooper RS, et al: Sex and race differences in sodium-lithium countertransport and red cell sodium concentration. Am J Epidemiol 120:537–541, 1984
Tupin JP, Schuller AB: Lithium and haloperidol incompatibility reviewed. Psychiatr J Univ Ottawa 3:1283–1287, 1978
Vestergoard P, Shou M, Thomsen K: Monitoring of patients in prophylactic lithium treatment: an assessment based on recent kidney studies. Br J Psychiatry 140:185–187, 1982
Wood AJJ, Zhou HH: Ethnic differences in drug disposition and responsiveness. Clin Pharmacokinet 20:1–24, 1991
Yang YY: Prophylactic efficacy of lithium and its effective plasma levels in Chinese bipolar patients. Acta Psychiatr Scand 71:171–175, 1985
Zakowska-Dabrowska T, Rybakowski J: Lithium-induced EEG changes: relation to lithium level in serum and red blood cells. Acta Psychiatr Scand 49:457–465, 1973

Chapter 7

Influence of Ethnicity on Reduced Haloperidol Concentrations in Blood

Tadanobu Inaba, Ph.D., Toshiyuki Someya, M.D., Morikazu Shibasaki, M.D., Siu-Wa Tang, M.D., and Saburo Takahashi, M.D.

Haloperidol (HAL) is a potent neuroleptic drug that is widely used. The chemical structure of HAL shows butyrophenone at one end and phenyl-piperidine at the other end. This lipophilic compound contains many functional groups that are susceptible to drug-metabolizing enzymes (Eddington and Young 1990; Forsman and Larsson 1978; Forsman et al. 1977; Oida et al. 1989; Pape 1981).

Therapeutic drug monitoring is important for many drugs. However, optimal plasma levels of neuroleptic drugs or therapeutic windows are not well established (Itoh et al. 1980; Moulin et al. 1982; Rubin et al. 1980). One of the complications arises because drug metabolites are often pharmacologically active. Plasma levels of the parent drug alone would not be sufficient, and monitoring of its metabolites is necessary (Chang et al. 1987; Ereshefsky et al. 1984; Shostak et al. 1987). Further complicating these issues is the increasing recognition of the complex contributions that interethnic variations of drug metabolism have on drug monitoring (Inaba 1989; Kalow 1991; Lin and Finder 1983; Lin et al. 1989; Lou 1990; Potkin et al. 1984; Someya et al. 1990).

When HAL was administered to treat psychiatric patients, a metabolite of HAL, reduced haloperidol (RHAL), was found to be consistently present in plasma. Although RHAL is a rather weak dopamine D_2 receptor antagonist and may not contribute

We wish to thank Agnes Bleiwas for critically reading the manuscript.

significantly to the clinical effects of HAL, its conversion to HAL in vivo and in vitro was reported to be quite substantial by Korpi and colleagues (1984, 1985) and later by several other research groups (Chang et al. 1991; Jann et al. 1990; Midha et al. 1989). Therefore, RHAL can act as a pro-drug or reservoir of HAL. Significant levels of RHAL as well as HAL were detected in brain samples obtained from patients treated with HAL (Korpi et al. 1984). The question remains whether RHAL was formed in the brain tissue and whether RHAL may even be converted back to HAL in the brain. With this in mind, we address three topics in this chapter: 1) biochemical characterization of HAL ketone reductase; 2) RHAL production in red blood cells (RBC); and 3) the plasma RHAL/HAL ratio (i.e., reductase versus oxidative enzymes and their ethnic differences).

HALOPERIDOL CARBONYL REDUCTASE

The phenone or carbonyl part of the HAL molecule has been known to be reduced to RHAL for some time (Forsman and Larsson 1978), but years passed before RHAL was measured in plasma of psychiatric patients. Biochemical studies had also been neglected. Rats have proven to be a poor model for reductases; fortunately, Korpi and colleagues (1985) discovered that the guinea pig was a suitable animal to use in the study of HAL reduction. Several reports (including ours) confirmed that guinea pigs are suitable for the reductase work (Chang et al. 1991; Eddington and Young 1990; Inaba and Kovacs 1989). Apparently Korpi's study described only very low concentration ranges of HAL and indicated that RHAL production was not nicotinamide adenine dinucleotide phosphate (NADPH)–dependent. The finding was rather puzzling for this type of reaction, because reduction pathways normally require electrons or reducing equivalents. It is likely that the endogenous NADPH concentration was sufficiently high when only low concentrations of HAL were used as done by this group.

Because liver is very rich in drug-metabolizing enzymes and a human liver bank was already set up at the University of Toronto some years ago, we initiated detailed biochemical studies of the reduction of HAL carbonyl group using human liver obtained from kidney donors. In contrast to the data by Korpi and colleagues (1985), the reduction of HAL was found to be dependent on NADPH (Inaba and Kovacs 1989). Although the cytosol fraction of the guinea pig liver was not investigated by Korpi and colleagues, we found abundant HAL reductase activity in both microsomes and cytosol of guinea pigs (Figure 7–1). In human liver, HAL reductase was detectable only in the cytosol and not in microsomes. One of the best ways to characterize an enzyme is by using various inhibitors. The potent inhibition of HAL reduction by well-known carbonyl reductase inhibitors, daunorubicin, ethacrynic acid, and menadione—but not by inhibitors of alcohol dehydrogenase and aldehyde dehydrogenase—strongly supported that the HAL reductase was a carbonyl reductase.

RHAL FORMATION IN BLOOD

Carbonyl reductases have not been investigated as fully as some other drug-metabolizing enzymes (e.g., cytochrome P_{450} and glucuronyltransferase). Nevertheless, reports in the literature in-

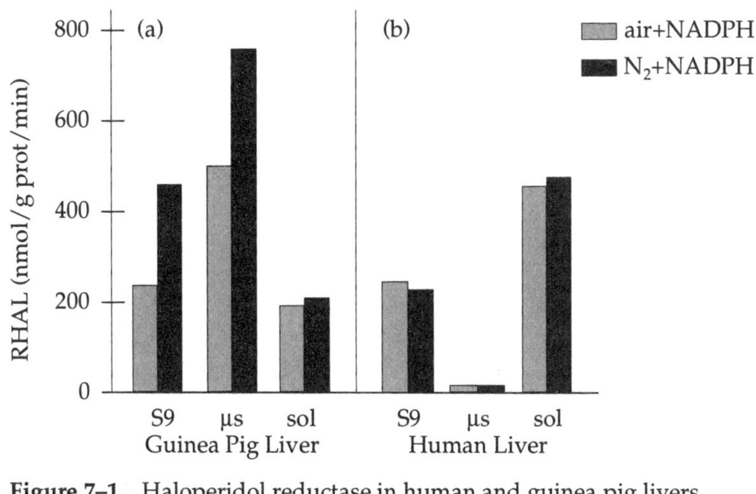

Figure 7–1. Haloperidol reductase in human and guinea pig livers (S9 = 9,000 g supernatant; μs = microsome; sol = cytosol; RHAL = reduced haloperidol; NADPH = nicotinamide adenine dinucleotide phosphate; N_2 = nitrogen).

dicated that carbonyl reductases were present in other tissues such as kidneys, RBC, and brain (Bachur 1976; Bohren et al. 1987; Cohen and Flockhart 1975; Wermuth et al. 1988). The tissue besides liver that had ample HAL carbonyl reductase activity was found to be RBC (Inaba et al. 1989; Someya et al. 1991). The inhibition pattern of HAL reductase in RBC was identical to the inhibition pattern in the liver.

Some researchers in psychiatry reported that RHAL concentrations were higher in RBC than in plasma (Ko et al. 1989; Volavka and Cooper 1987). However, no one had previously suggested that RHAL was produced in this tissue. Some investigators attempted to utilize HAL concentrations in RBC rather than plasma to improve drug therapy (Neborsky et al. 1982; Smith et al. 1985). The fact that RHAL concentrations are higher in RBC than in plasma and that HAL concentrations are similar in both tissues can be visualized in Figure 7–2, where RBC/plasma ratios of RHAL and HAL were plotted. It is evident that the individual variation is large and that RHAL showed higher

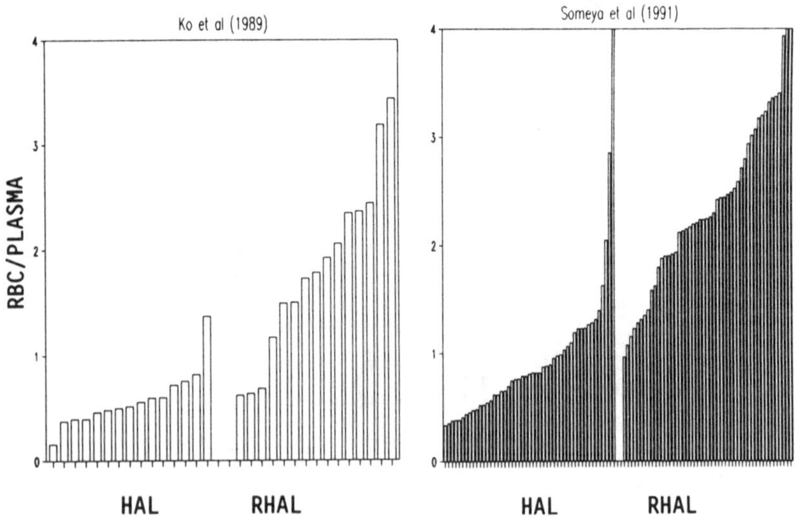

Figure 7–2. RBC/plasma ratios of HAL and RHAL. *Left panel:* plotted from data of Ko et al. 1989 (n = 15); *right panel:* plotted from data of Shibasaki et al., in press (n = 49). (RBC = red blood cells; HAL = haloperidol; RHAL = reduced haloperidol.)

RBC/plasma ratios than 1, indicating high affinity for RBC. The ethnic origin of patients in the study by Ko and colleagues was not stated, but most patients in New York are likely to be non-Asians. The data from Japanese patients ($n = 49$; Shibasaki et al., in press) are included for comparison in this figure, and there was little or no ethnic difference.

RHAL/HAL IN PLASMA

The use of plasma RHAL/HAL ratios rather than HAL concentrations for therapeutic drug monitoring was first advocated by Ereshefsky et al. (1984). Usually plasma HAL levels are reported to be linearly dose-dependent (Itoh et al. 1980; Matsuno et al. 1990; Moulin et al. 1982). However, in spite of efforts to establish a therapeutic window, the dosage of HAL must be titrated to an individual's need. A different index rather than plasma HAL levels was sought, and RHAL/HAL ratios have been proposed. Although only five patients were studied by Ereshefsky and colleagues (1984), it was nonetheless clear that the RHAL/HAL ratio was independent of the dose and might be a useful index. The observation of an independent relation between the ratio and the dose was also confirmed in a larger group of patients ($n = 45$, Someya et al. 1990) in a different ethnic group.

Until recently, the difficulty in recruiting large numbers of patients resulted in the lack of studies of the pharmacogenetics of HAL and population analysis. The first such investigation was made by Someya and colleagues (1990) in Japanese patients, where a nonnormal or likely bimodal distribution of plasma RHAL/HAL ratios was observed. The antimode appeared to be 0.7; most Chinese and Japanese patients were below this value, whereas most Caucasian patients showed higher ratios (Table 7–1). The data for other ethnic groups were obtained from various reports and plotted in Figure 7–3—the data on Caucasians from Altamura and colleagues (1988) and Ko and colleagues (1989), and the data on Asians from Chang and colleagues (1989) and Shibasaki and colleagues (in press; $n = 79$).

The RHAL/HAL ratio can be influenced by either the numerator or the denominator or by both. In other words, not only the reductase but also the reverse process, the oxidative pathway, can influence the ratio. Earlier work by Korpi and colleagues (1985) using guinea pig liver suggested the involvement of cytochrome P_{450} in the reduction of HAL. Additional evidence for the involvement of P_{450} came from the observation in which HAL was recognized as a potent inhibitor of the polymorphic human P_{450}, debrisoquine hydroxylase (CYP2D6). It was surprising that RHAL was even a more potent inhibitor, indicating high affinity for this particular cytochrome P_{450} enzyme (Tyndale et al. 1991). Microsomal oxidation of RHAL to HAL was demonstrated in human liver. The reaction was stereoselectively inhibited by quinidine and its stereoisomer, quinine, which are the most useful pair of inhibitors to characterize debrisoquine hydroxylase. Less selectivity shown for RHAL as a substrate suggested that other enzymes may be involved.

The defective debrisoquine hydroxylase occurs in 6%–8% of Caucasians and about 1% of Asians. Slow metabolizers of debrisoquine/sparteine would not convert RHAL to HAL, perhaps requiring higher HAL doses. Besides the frequency differ-

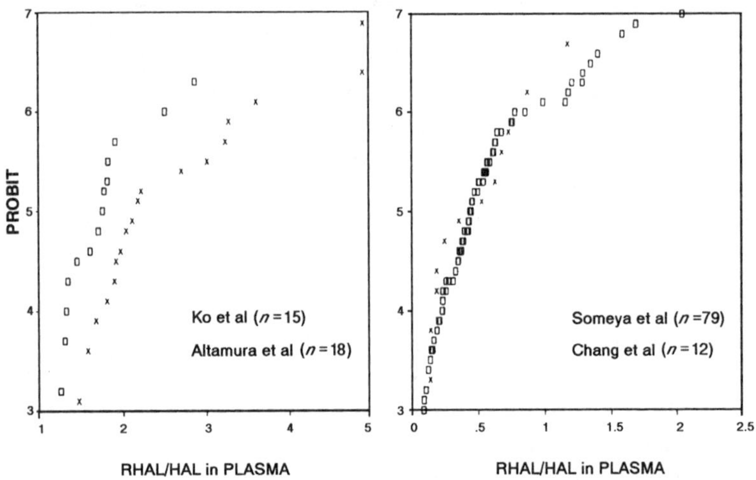

Figure 7–3. Plasma RHAL/HAL ratios in Caucasians and Asians. *Left panel:* data on Caucasian subjects from Ko et al. 1989 (n = 15) and Altamura et al. 1988 (n = 18); *right panel:* data on Asian subjects from Chang et al. 1989 (n = 12) and Shibasaki et al., in press (n = 79). (RHAL/HAL = reduced haloperidol/haloperidol.)

Table 7–1. Ethnic variability of RHAL/HAL in plasma

Ethnic origin	RHAL/HAL (mean)	Frequency (high/low[a][%])	Reference
Caucasian (n = 5)	2.13	80 / 20	Ereshefsky et al. 1984
Caucasian (n = 18)	1.91	83 / 17	Altamura et al. 1988
Caucasian (n = 15)	0.86	60 / 40	Ko et al. 1989
Chinese (n = 21)	0.31	0 / 100	Chang et al. 1987
Japanese (n = 79)	0.55	19 / 81	Shibayashi et al., in press

Note. RHAL/HAL = reduced haloperidol/haloperidol.
[a] Antimode RHAL/HAL = 0.7.

ence of slow debrisoquine metabolizers between Caucasians and Asians, in general, Caucasians oxidize or hydroxylate drugs faster than their Asian counterparts. Although we have no appropriate probe drugs to assess an individual's carbonyl reductase activity, the difference in plasma RHAL/HAL ratios between Caucasians and Asians (Table 7–1) may be affected predominantly by oxidation.

In summary, the plasma ratio RHAL/HAL in patients regularly treated with HAL still showed no clear-cut relation with the clinical effect. Some other factor or other metabolic pathway may be involved to further complicate and prevent us from establishing the therapeutic window. The cause of the ethnic difference in the RHAL/HAL ratios mentioned previously still needs to be resolved.

REFERENCES

Altamura C, Mauri M, Cavallaro R, et al: Reduced haloperidol/haloperidol ratio and clinical outcome in schizophrenia. Prog Neuropsychopharmacol Biol Psychiatry 12:689–694, 1988

Bachur NR: Cytoplasmic aldo-keto reductases: a class of drug metabolizing enzymes. Science 93:595–597, 1976

Bohren KM, von Wartburg JP, Wermuth B: Kinetics of carbonyl reductase from human brain. Biochem J 244:165–171, 1987

Chang WH, Chen TY, Lee CF, et al: Low plasma reduced haloperidol/haloperidol ratios in Chinese patients. Biol Psychiatry 22:1406–1408, 1987

Chang WH, Lin SK, Jann MW, et al: Pharmacodynamics and pharmacokinetics of haloperidol and reduced haloperidol in schizophrenic patients. Biol Psychiatry 26:239–249, 1989
Chang WH, Lin KS, Jann MW: Interconversions between haloperidol and reduced haloperidol in schizophrenic patients and guinea pigs. J Clin Psychopharmacol 11:99–105, 1991
Cohen GM, Flockhart IR: The partial purification and properties of a human erythrocyte 4-nitroacetophenone reductase. Xenobiotica 5:213–222, 1975
Eddington ND, Young D: Biliary excretion of reduced haloperidol glucuronide. Psychopharmacology (Berlin) 100:46–48, 1990
Ereshefsky L, Davis CM, Harrington CA, et al: Haloperidol and reduced haloperidol plasma levels in selected schizophrenic patients. J Clin Psychopharmacol 4:138–142, 1984
Forsman A, Larsson M: Metabolism of haloperidol. Current Therapeutic Research and Clinical Experimentation 24:567–569, 1978
Forsman A, Folsch G, Larsson M, et al: On the metabolism of haloperidol in man. Current Therapeutic Research and Clinical Experimentation 21:606–617, 1977
Inaba T: Pharmacogenetic polymorphism: mephenytoin hydroxylation deficiency, in Xenobiotic Metabolism and Disposition. Edited by Kato R, Estabrook RW, Cayen MN. London, Taylor & Francis, 1989, pp 467–474
Inaba T, Kovacs J: Haloperidol reductase in human and guinea pig livers. Drug Metab Dispos 17:330–333, 1989
Inaba T, Kalow W, Someya T, et al: Haloperidol reduction can be assayed in human red blood cells. Can J Physiol Pharmacol 67:1468–1469, 1989
Itoh H, Yagi G, Ohtsuka N, et al: Serum level of haloperidol and its clinical significance. Prog Neuropsychopharmacol Biol Psychiatry 4:171–183, 1980
Jann MW, Lam YWF, Chang WH: Reversible metabolism of haloperidol and reduced haloperidol in Chinese schizophrenic patients. Psychopharmacology (Berlin) 101:107–111, 1990
Kalow W: Interethnic variation of drug metabolism. Trends Pharmacol Sci 12:102–107, 1991
Ko GN, Korpi ER, Kirch DG: Haloperidol and reduced haloperidol concentrations in plasma and red blood cells from chronic schizophrenic patients. J Clin Psychopharmacol 9:186–190, 1989
Korpi ER, Kleinman JE, Costakos DT, et al: Reduced haloperidol in the post-mortem brains of haloperidol-treated patients. Psychiatry Res 11:259–269, 1984

Korpi ER, Costakos DT, Wyatt RJ: Interconversion of haloperidol and reduced haloperidol in guinea pig and rat liver microsomes. Biochem Pharmacol 34:2923–2927, 1985

Lin KM, Finder E: Neuroleptic dosage for Asians. Am J Psychiatry 140:490–491, 1983

Lin KM, Poland RE, Nuccio I, et al: Longitudinal assessment of haloperidol doses and serum concentrations in Asian and Caucasian schizophrenic patients. Am J Psychiatry 146:1307–1311, 1989

Lou YC: Differences in drug metabolism polymorphism between Orientals and Caucasians. Drug Metab Rev 22:451–475, 1990

Matsuno H, Uematsu T, Nakashima M: The measurement of haloperidol and reduced haloperidol in hair as an index of dosage history. Br J Clin Pharmacol 29:187–194, 1990

Midha KK, Chakraborty BS, Ganes DA, et al: Intersubject variation in the pharmacokinetics of haloperidol and reduced haloperidol. J Clin Psychopharmacol 9:98–104, 1989

Moulin MA, Davy JP, Debruyne D, et al: Serum level monitoring and therapeutic effect of haloperidol in schizophrenic patients. Psychopharmacology (Berlin) 76:346–350, 1982

Neborsky R, Janowsky DS, Perel J, et al: Haloperidol plasma/red blood cell ratios and clinical efficacy. Psychopharmacol Bull 18:17–20, 1982

Oida T, Terauchi Y, Toshida K, et al: Use of antisera in the isolation of human specific conjugates of haloperidol. Xenobiotica 19:781–793, 1989

Pape BE: Isolation and identification of a metabolite of haloperidol. J Anal Toxicol 5:113–117, 1981

Potkin SG, Shen Y, Pardes H, et al: Haloperidol concentrations elevated in Chinese patients. Psychiatry Res 12:167–172, 1984

Rubin RT, Forsman A, Heykants J, et al: Serum haloperidol determinations in psychiatric patients. Arch Gen Psychiatry 37:1069–1074, 1980

Shibasaki M, Someya T, Takahashi S: Relation of red blood cells' reduced haloperidol concentrations to haloperidol reductase activity assayed in red blood cells in psychiatric patients. Prog Neuropsychopharmacol Biol Psychiatry (in press)

Shostak M, Perel JM, Stiller RL, et al: Plasma haloperidol and clinical response: a role for reduced haloperidol in antipsychotic activity. J Clin Psychopharmacol 7:394–400, 1987

Smith RC, Baumgartner R, Shvartsburd A, et al: Comparative efficacy of red cell and plasma haloperidol as predictors of clinical response in schizophrenics. Psychopharmacology (Berlin) 85:449–455, 1985

Someya T, Takahashi S, Shibasaki M, et al: Reduced haloperidol/haloperidol ratios in plasma: polymorphism in Japanese psychiatric patients. Psychiatry Res 31:111–120, 1990

Someya T, Shibasaki M, Kato T, et al: Haloperidol reductase activity in red blood cells from Oriental patients on haloperidol. Prog Neuropsychopharmacol Biol Psychiatry 14:941–947, 1991

Tyndale RF, Kalow W, Inaba T: Oxidation of reduced haloperidol to haloperidol: involvement of human P450IID6 (sparteine/debrisoquine monooxygenase). Br J Clin Pharmacol 31:655–660, 1991

Volavka J, Cooper TB: Review of haloperidol blood levels and clinical response: looking through the window. J Clin Psychopharmacol 7:25–30, 1987

Wermuth B, Bohren KM, Heinemann G, et al: Human carbonyl reductase. J Biol Chem 263:16185–16188, 1988

Chapter 8

Haloperidol and Reduced Haloperidol Plasma Concentrations in Different Ethnic Populations and Interindividual Variabilities in Haloperidol Metabolism

Michael W. Jann, Pharm.D.,
Y. W. Francis Lam, Pharm.D.,
and Wen-Ho Chang, M.D.

Ethnicity has been suggested to play a key role in the metabolism of various psychotropic agents. The biological basis for ethnic variability in drug metabolism could be related to the enzymes and genes that determine the pattern of metabolism (Kalow 1982). Diversity in the enzyme quantity, molecular structure, and biochemical modifiers of enzyme activity can be possible sources of variation that clinical observations cannot accurately assess (Kalow 1982). Examples of drug metabolic differences between Chinese and Caucasian populations were reported with tricyclic antidepressants (Kalow et al. 1980; Rudorfer et al. 1984, 1985) and codeine (Yue et al. 1989).

For neuroleptic agents, several investigators have reported that lower neuroleptic dosages are observed in Asian populations compared to Caucasians (Lin and Finder 1983). However, this finding was not observed by other researchers (Sramek et al. 1986). The incidence of extrapyramidal side effects (EPS) also was

Supported by grant NSC 79-412-B109-01 from the National Science Council and Taipei City Government, Taiwan, Republic of China. Presented at the American Psychiatric Association Annual Meeting, New Orleans, LA, May 1991.

reported to be higher in Asian groups compared to African-American and Caucasian patients treated with haloperidol (HAL; Binder and Levy 1981). In a fixed dose study of HAL with age-matched groups ($N = 18$), Potkin and colleagues (1984) reported 52% higher HAL serum concentrations in Chinese compared to Caucasian psychiatric patients. In a single fixed dose of HAL given intramuscularly or orally, Caucasians had lower serum HAL and prolactin concentrations compared to American-born and foreign-born Asians (Lin et al. 1988). A longitudinal evaluation of HAL doses and serum concentrations showed that Asians experienced a higher episode of EPS and serum concentrations compared to Caucasians (K. M. Lin et al. 1989).

The pharmacokinetics of HAL in humans has been extensively studied (Cheng et al. 1987; Forsman and Ohman 1976; Holley et al. 1983). HAL's metabolic profile involves N-dealkylation and the formation of piperidine and 4-fluorobenzoylpropionic acid metabolites (Forsman et al. 1977). Reduction of the benzylic ketone C=O group to C—OH forming the reduced metabolite reduced haloperidol (RHAL) has been suggested to be the other major metabolic route (Froemming et al. 1989). In 1978, Forsman and Larsson reported equal plasma concentrations of RHAL and HAL in psychiatric patients. Some investigations have suggested that elevated RHAL concentrations are associated with a diminished therapeutic response to HAL (Altamura et al. 1988; Ereshefsky et al. 1984) or play a significant role in antipsychotic activity and therefore should not be neglected (Shostak et al. 1987).

HAL has been shown to be converted to RHAL in the guinea pig model (Korpi et al. 1985a, 1985b). The enzyme responsible for this conversion has been determined to be HAL reductase (Inaba and Kovacs 1989). This enzyme was found in hepatic tissues in both humans and guinea pigs. Kirch and colleagues (1985a) demonstrated in electrophysiological experiments that RHAL lacked neuroleptic activity. However, RHAL stimulated prolactin levels greater than clozapine and thioridazine but less than HAL (Hays et al. 1980). RHAL had approximately one-third to one-fifth the potency of HAL in producing elevations of homovanillic acid (HVA) levels in rat prefrontal cortex and caudate (Bowen et al. 1990; Chang et al. 1987a, 1987b). In receptor binding affinity, RHAL had an 85-fold lower binding affinity compared to HAL at the D_2 receptor but an equal affinity at the sigma opiate receptor (Bowen et al. 1990). RHAL was reported to be one-fifth as potent as HAL in inhibiting apomorphine-induced stereotypy in rats (Browning et al. 1982). RHAL is oxidized back to HAL in humans and thus HAL metabolism follows a reduction/oxidation cycle or interconversion process as shown in Figure 8–1 (Chakraborty et al. 1989; Jann et al. 1990). Variations in the interconversion process and the N-dealkylation pathways could account for the wide interpatient variability observed within each ethnic group.

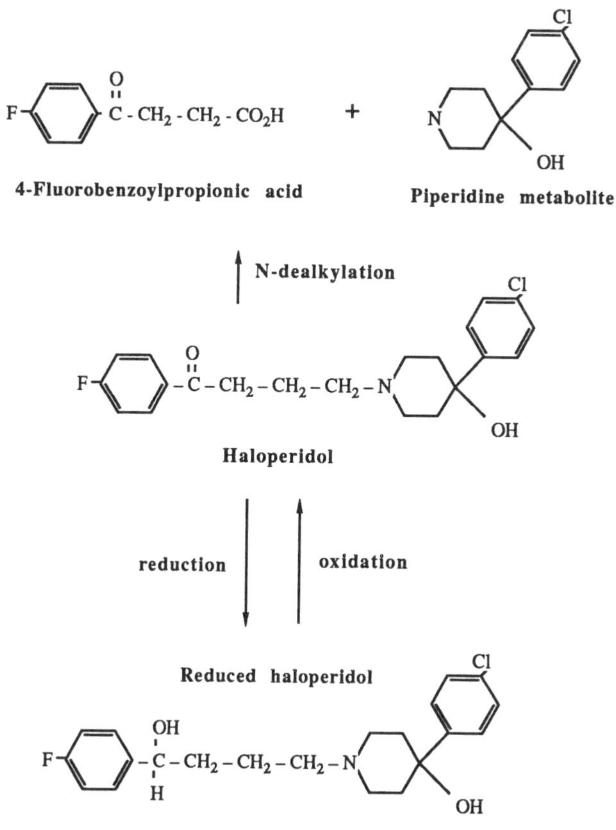

Figure 8–1. Metabolic pathways of haloperidol.

HAL and RHAL plasma concentrations have been reported in various ethnic groups (Chang et al. 1987c; Jann et al. 1989; Midha et al. 1989; Someya et al. 1989). RHAL was detected in only 6 of 28 control subjects given a single 5-mg HAL dose (Midha et al. 1989). The reduced metabolite level was generally much lower than HAL. In Chinese psychiatric patients treated with HAL 20 mg/day for 6 weeks, RHAL plasma levels were three- to fourfold lower than HAL plasma levels (Chang et al. 1987c). Two different ratios (high versus low) of RHAL to HAL were reported among Japanese patients (Someya et al. 1989). In comparing Chinese with non-Chinese groups, although HAL plasma concentrations did not differ, RHAL was shown to be threefold lower in Chinese patients (Jann et al. 1989). This study will further extend our investigation of possible ethnic differences in HAL and RHAL plasma concentrations and examine the reversible metabolic process investigating interindividual variations within an ethnic group.

METHODS

Part I—Analysis of HAL and RHAL Plasma Levels

Chinese psychiatric patients ($n = 156$) were hospitalized at the Taipei City Psychiatric Center, Military Psychiatric Center, and National Taiwan University Hospital (Jann et al. 1992). The remaining Caucasian ($n = 37$), Hispanic ($n = 51$), and African-American ($n = 23$) patients were hospitalized at the San Antonio State Hospital. All Chinese and non-Chinese patients were diagnosed as schizophrenic according to DSM-III criteria (American Psychiatric Association 1980). Medical histories and laboratory data (SMA 12/60, urinalysis, hematology, serology, and electrolytes) were collected from each patient. All laboratory parameters were within normal limits. Schizophrenic patients were selected for comparative analysis based upon the following parameters: stable HAL dosage for a minimum of 7 days; no enzyme inducing agents (e.g., phenobarbital) or inhibiting drugs (e.g., cimetidine); nonsmokers or persons who smoked less than one pack per day of cigarettes (usually approximately half a pack); no oral or intramuscular HAL administered prn 48 hours prior to serum sampling; and steady-state HAL serum concentrations obtained at each dosage.

HAL used in Taiwan and San Antonio was purchased from Janssen Pharmaceuticals in Beerse, Belgium, and McNeil Pharmaceuticals in Spring House, Pennsylvania. The HAL dosages for both non-Chinese and Chinese patients were individually titrated based on clinical response. The only concurrent medications allowed were benztropine and trihexyphenidyl, which do not influence HAL serum concentrations (Itoh et al. 1980; Linniola et al. 1980). Clinical assessments made by each clinician were without utilization of a standardized rating scale but based on patient interviews, patient-to-patient interactions, and unit staff and nursing information. The incidence of EPS could not be assessed with validity because of the prophylactic use of anticholinergic medications in some patients. Therefore, comparative analysis was not attempted for clinical response and adverse effects.

HAL and RHAL blood samples were obtained 10–12 hours after the evening dose and prior to the morning dose. Samples in non-Chinese ethnic groups were centrifuged, and plasma specimens were sent to the University of Texas Mental Science Institute (UTMSI) for analysis. Blood samples from Chinese subjects were centrifuged and plasma stored at –60°C until assay. RHAL and HAL assayed by UTMSI utilized a combined liquid chromatography and radioimmunoassay (LC/RIA) method without cross-reactivity to other metabolites (Browning et al. 1985). The lower limit of the assay is less than 1 ng/ml, with intra-assay and interassay coefficients of variation less than 10% for RHAL and HAL at 5–10 ng/ml. Plasma HAL and RHAL samples from Chinese subjects were assayed via reverse phase liquid chromatography (LC) with electrochemical detection (Chang et al. 1989; Korpi et al. 1983). The minimum level of sensitivity was 0.4 ng/ml, with intra-assay and interassay coefficients of variation from 4%–12% at 2–10 ng/ml. The UTMSI set up the identical LC technique used in Chinese patients and compared identical patient samples with LC and LC/RIA assay methods in which the correlation coefficients for HAL and RHAL were $r = 0.96$ ($P < .02$) and $r = 0.98$ ($P < .01$), respectively.

Statistical analysis comparing demographic data, HAL dosages, and HAL and RHAL plasma levels was completed by SAS that utilized paired and unpaired Student's *t* test, two-way analysis of covariance (ANCOVA), and linear regression analysis with Pearson Product correlation coefficient. A Stepwise Multiple Regression Model (General Linear Models Procedure) was used to determine which factors could influence HAL plasma levels (SAS Institute 1985). Significance levels of $P < .05$ were considered statistically significant.

Part II—Variabilities in Interindividual HAL Metabolism

Seven Chinese male schizophrenic patients (diagnosed using DSM-III-R [American Psychiatric Association 1987]) were recruited for this phase of the study. The subjects' mean age was 29.4 ± 9.2 years, and their mean weight was 60.3 ± 7.6 kg. After obtaining informed consent, the subjects were given 0.5 mg/kg HAL or RHAL in a randomized crossover manner separated by a 2-week interval. They had not received prior oral neuroleptics for 4 weeks or depot neuroleptics for 4 months. A drug was given at 9:00 A.M., and blood samples were obtained at baseline and at 0.25, 0.5, 1.0, 1.5, 2.0, 2.5, 3.0, 3.5, 4, 4.5, 5, 6, 8, 12, 24, 36, 48, and 72 hours after drug administration. Four weeks after this phase was completed, the subjects were given HAL (10 mg bid) for the next 4 weeks. A weekly blood sample was obtained prior to the morning dose. The assay method has been described previously.

The kinetic parameters of HAL and RHAL from the single-dose study were determined for each subject. The area under the curve (AUC) was calculated by the log trapezoidal rule. When RHAL is converted back to HAL, the clearance (CL) of HAL is dependent not only on its own elimination rate but also on the elimination rate of RHAL. Using the model that has been used for predisone/prednisone, the metabolic process for the N-dealkylation, interconversion, and glucuronidation can be determined (Lam et al. 1992; see Figure 8–2).

The interconversion of HAL and RHAL CL is represented by $CL_{1,2}$ and $CL_{2,1}$. The N-dealkylation pathway for HAL is represented by $CL_{1,0}$ and the glucuronidation route of RHAL by $CL_{2,0}$. The total oral CL for HAL is the sum of $CL_{1,0}$ and $CL_{1,2}$. Similarly, total CL for RHAL is the sum of $CL_{2,0}$ and $CL_{2,1}$. Each CL param-

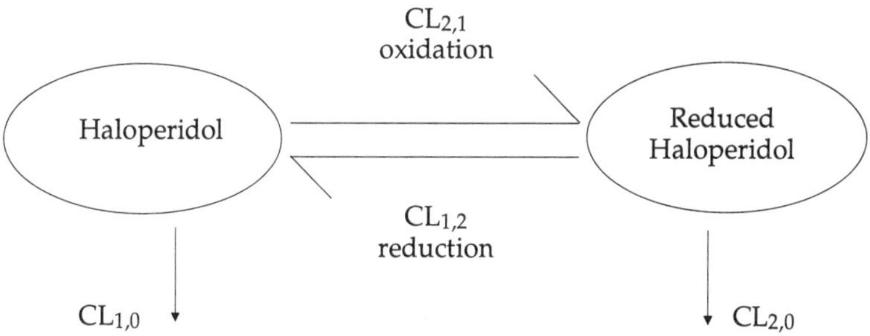

Figure 8–2. Pharmacokinetic model for interconversion of haloperidol and reduced haloperidol.

eter can be calculated by utilizing previous mathematical formulas between dose and AUC for HAL and RHAL (Jann et al. 1990).

RESULTS

Part I

Comparisons between each non-Chinese ethnic group versus the Chinese group are also shown in Table 8–1. The African-American group was significantly older ($t = 3.05$, df = 177, $P < .005$) and weighed more ($t = 2.29$, df = 177, $P = .031$) than the Chinese group. The HAL daily dose did differ significantly between the two groups ($t = 2.57$, df = 177, $P = .017$), but there was no significant difference in HAL plasma levels between the two groups ($t = 0.54$, df = 177, $P = .596$). The African-American group had higher RHAL plasma levels ($t = 2.04$, df = 177, $P = .043$), whereas the Chinese group had RHAL/HAL ratios that were significantly lower ($t = 3.39$, df = 177, $P = .003$). This profile also was observed with the Caucasian group, as significantly older ages, greater weight, and higher HAL doses were found ($t = 6.02$, df = 191, $P < .001$; $t = 3.86$, df = 191, $P < .001$; $t = 2.83$, df = 191, $P = .007$, respectively). However, plasma HAL levels did not differ ($t = 0.38$, df = 191, $P = .704$). Again, RHAL plasma concentrations were higher in the Caucasian group and ratios of RHAL/HAL were lower in the Chinese group ($t = 2.22$, df = 191, $P = .028$; $t = 4.34$, df = 4.34, $P < .001$). The Hispanic group, when compared to the Chinese group, had consistently significantly higher values in all five parameters ($P < .005$), including HAL dose and plasma concentrations.

Analysis between the non-Chinese ethnic groups showed that the Caucasian and African-American groups had no significant differences in HAL and RHAL plasma levels, RHAL/HAL ratios, and HAL dosage. The Hispanic group differed from both Caucasian and African-American groups in all those parameters, but the HAL daily dose and HAL plasma concentrations for this group were also significantly higher than both other groups ($t = 2.01$, df = 72, $P = .048$; $t = 2.84$, df = 86, $P < .01$, respectively).

The relationship between HAL daily dose (mg/day) and plasma concentrations (ng/ml) for the various ethnic populations is shown in Figure 8–3A. The correlation coefficients for each ethnic group were as follows: Chinese ($r^2 = 0.396$, df = 1,151, $F = 46.614$, $P < .001$); African-American ($r^2 = 0.801$, df = 1,21, $F = 84.611$, $P < .001$); Hispanic ($r^2 = 0.486$, df = 1,46, $F = 43.505$, $P < .001$); and Caucasian ($r^2 = 0.716$, df = 1,35, $F = 88.469$, $P < .001$). Each ethnic group had a large interpatient variation in HAL plasma levels at the same dose. The Chinese group displays a distinct difference compared to the remaining ethnic groups.

Table 8–1. Summary of patient demographics, haloperidol, and reduced haloperidol parameters (mean ± SD)

Ethnic group	*N*	Age (yrs)	Wt (kg)	HAL dose (mg/day)	HAL Cp (ng/ml)	RHAL Cp (ng/ml)	RHAL/HAL ratio
Chinese	156	29.9 ±9.4	55.8 ±7.9	21.1 ±12.9	18.3 ±13.4	11.4 ±18.9	0.48 ±0.41
Caucasian	37	45.1 ±14.6	69.8[a] ±21.7	33.1[a,b] ±25.1	17.2[b] ±15.9	19.6[a] ±24.5	0.95[a] ±0.59
Hispanic	51	40.1[a] ±10.4	71.1[a] ±16.7	471[a,b] ±22.0	28.4[a,b] ±22.5	33.4[a] ±46.1	1.04[a] ±0.59
African-American	23	39.8[a] ±15.1	64.8[a] ±18.5	35.5[a,b] ±26.5	16.4[b] ±15.8	20.5[a] ±26.3	0.97[a] ±0.66

Note. C_p = plasma concentration; HAL = haloperidol; RHAL = reduced haloperidol.

[a] $P < .01$, Chinese versus Caucasian, Chinese versus African-American, and Chinese versus Hispanic.

[b] $P < .05$, Caucasian versus Hispanic and African-American versus Hispanic.

The African-American and Caucasian groups appear to have a parallel line, whereas the Hispanic group does not appear to diverge until HAL dosages greater than 40 mg/day are achieved.

The relationship between HAL and RHAL plasma levels (ng/ml) for the different ethnic groups is shown in Figure 8–3B.

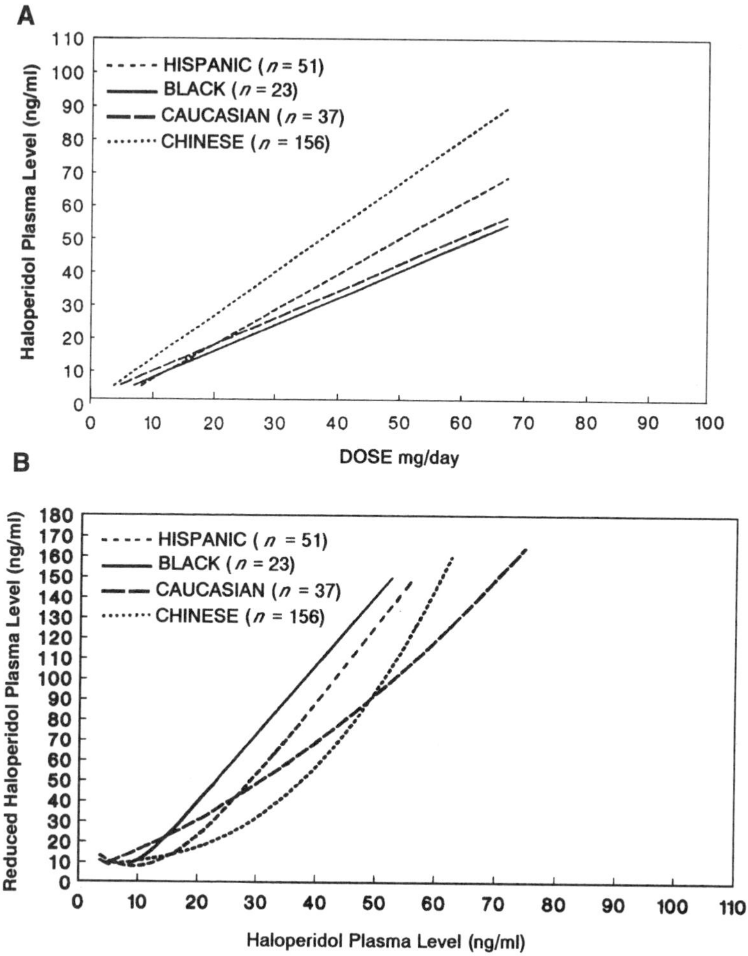

Figure 8–3. Comparison of haloperidol (*A*) and reduced haloperidol (*B*) plasma levels in different ethnic groups. Reprinted with permission from Jann et al. 1992.

Inspection of the graphic plots for the different ethnic populations reveals a nonlinear relationship between RHAL and HAL plasma concentrations. This figure demonstrates distinct differences between each ethnic group regarding HAL and RHAL plasma level relationships. The Chinese group has the lowest RHAL concentration for a given plasma concentration of HAL ratios until a concentration of approximately 50 ng/ml of HAL is reached. At that point, a more dramatic increase in RHAL plasma levels takes place. In the African-American population, the RHAL plasma level relationship appears to be the highest when compared to the other ethnic groups. The relationship between RHAL and HAL plasma concentrations in the Hispanic group resembles that of the African-American group only in that the curve is shifted to the right, with a rapid rise in RHAL plasma levels when HAL plasma concentrations exceed 30 ng/ml. In the Caucasian group, the increase in RHAL plasma levels with the increase in HAL plasma levels are modest even when HAL plasma concentrations exceed 40 ng/ml.

The stepwise multiple regression analysis evaluated eight variables that could possibly influence HAL plasma concentrations. As shown in Table 8–2, the factors that were found to be statistically significant include dose, RHAL concentrations, and Chinese and African-American populations. When these eight factors were combined together, a correlation of $r^2 = 0.74$, df = 6, 260, $F = 126.012$, $P < .001$ was calculated. The African-American group had only a $P = .0546$; but based on the various data from

Table 8–2. Stepwise regression analysis of factors influencing haloperidol serum concentrations

Factor	F value	P value
Dose	11.153	< .001
RHAL Cp	9.553	< .001
Chinese	3.093	.002
African-American	1.931	.0546
Weight	1.641	.1019
Age	1.348	.1788
Caucasian	0.722	.4710
Hispanic	0.722	.4710

Note. RHAL Cp = reduced haloperidol plasma concentration.

the dose to RHAL plasma levels and RHAL to HAL plasma concentration relationships, this ethnic group most likely can be a significant factor influencing HAL plasma levels. Weight and age appear not to be significant factors in these populations. Interestingly, the Caucasian and Hispanic groups seem to have an analogous effect on the regression model. This could possibly suggest that Hispanic and Caucasian populations have a similar but not identical metabolic disposition for HAL.

Part II

The data investigating the interindividual metabolic variations within the same ethnic group are shown in Table 8–3, wherein 7 Chinese schizophrenic patients received HAL (10 mg bid) for 28 days. Each of these patients also received a single 0.5-mg/kg dose of HAL and RHAL, and the different metabolic clearances were determined for the interconversion and conversion pathways. The RHAL concentrations in patients 1 and 2 are lower than the others, whereas patient 3 had the highest plasma level. The individual CL values for the different metabolic pathways

Table 8–3. Haloperidol and reduced haloperidol plasma concentrations after 4 weeks of haloperidol dosing

Subject	Steady-state HAL conc.	Steady-state RHAL conc. (ng/ml)	RHAL/HAL ratio	$CL_{1,0}$	$CL_{2,0}$	$CL_{1,2}$	$CL_{2,1}$
1	19.5	4.4	0.23	0.82	0.19	0.06	0.06
2	18.7	4.6	0.38	1.17	0.16	0.32	0.44
3	20.0	12.9	0.39	0.05	0.48	0.34	0.11
4	18.0	6.0	0.31	0.69	0.70	0.41	0.52
5	18.4	5.7	0.31	0.71	0.24	0.32	0.31
6	11.3	6.3	0.56	1.05	0.47	0.62	0.32
7	15.4	7.2	0.47	0.70	0.32	0.53	0.46
Mean ± SD	17.3 ± 3.0	6.7 ±2.9	0.40 ±0.16	0.74 ±0.36	0.37 ±0.20	0.35 ±0.19	0.32 ±0.18

Note. 10-mg doses twice a day and clearance calculations of the metabolic conversions and interconversions of HAL and RHAL after a single 0.5-mg/kg dose of HAL and RHAL. CL = clearance (L/kg/hour); $CL_{1,0}$ = N-dealkylation pathway; $CL_{2,0}$ = glucuronidation pathway; $CL_{1,2}$ = reduction pathway; $CL_{2,1}$ = oxidation pathway; HAL = haloperidol; RHAL = reduced haloperidol.

are also presented in Table 8–3. The RHAL/HAL ratio was obtained on day 28. The mean metabolic rates for reduction and oxidation are almost identical. However, there was an eight- to tenfold variation for reduction and oxidation between these patients. The reduction of HAL to RHAL and its back oxidation in patient 1 was extremely small. Patient 3 also displayed a small oxidative capacity, but the reduction clearance was similar to that of the remaining patients.

Variabilities in the elimination pathways of HAL and RHAL in the N-dealkylation ($CL_{1,0}$) and glucuronidation ($CL_{2,0}$) routes were also observed. Patient 3 had the lowest elimination rate of 0.05 L/kg/hour that was at least 14 times lower than that of the other patients. The diminished capacity in this pathway can account for the low total HAL clearance. An approximate variation for RHAL of 4.5-fold was observed in all patients. A plot of RHAL/HAL ratios versus the reduction clearance of HAL to RHAL is shown in Figure 8–3B. Although a positive correlation was found, the data suggest that the ratio is only partially related to the reductive capacity.

The mean total clearance for HAL ($CL_{1,0} + CL_{1,2}$) and RHAL ($CL_{2,0} + CL_{2,1}$) was 1.09 ± 0.43 L/kg/hour and 0.68 ± 0.30 L/kg/hour, respectively. These CL values are similar to those previously reported by us in another group of Chinese schizophrenic patients who were given a smaller HAL dose (Jann et al. 1990).

DISCUSSION

These results describe the variations in HAL and RHAL plasma levels in different ethnic populations and interindividual differences within an ethnic group. Previous investigations have reported differences in HAL doses and plasma concentrations between Chinese and Caucasian subjects (K. M. Lin et al. 1988, 1989; Potkin et al. 1984) and other non-Chinese ethnic groups (Jann et al. 1989). This chapter supports these earlier findings. Although considerable interpatient variability within each ethnic group exists between HAL dose and plasma levels, the regression line for the Chinese group differs from the remaining ethnic populations shown in Figure 8–3A. For example, at 20 mg/day, the regression lines for the non-Chinese groups are clustered together but distinctly separate from the Chinese population. The corresponding HAL plasma concentrations are approximately 40%–50% higher in Chinese patients compared to non-Chinese patients. This approximation would also support previous investigations (Potkin et al. 1984). With dosages higher than 40 mg/day, the Hispanic group also had a higher HAL plasma concentration. The African-American and Caucasian groups share an almost-identical profile, except that the regression line is shifted slightly to the right for the African-American group. However, the African-American group had the smallest number of patients; with a larger population, a larger interpatient variability might have occurred.

Dosing information for HAL can also be implied from Figure 8–3A. If most investigators suggest that the upper therapeutic limit or plateau for HAL plasma concentrations is roughly 20–25 ng/ml (Kirch et al. 1985b; Volavka and Cooper 1987), then dosages greater than 30 mg/day would not be necessary in Chinese patients. HAL dosages greater than 50–60 mg/day might not be needed in non-Chinese patients.

The HAL plasma concentrations among the Chinese, Caucasian, and African-American groups did not significantly differ in clinical settings. However, the HAL dosages required for the Caucasian and African-American groups were significantly greater than what was needed for the Chinese group to achieve comparable plasma levels. This finding further supports previous reports (Jann et al. 1989). RHAL plasma levels and RHAL/HAL ratios were considerably lower in the Chinese population. Direct comparisons with the Hispanic group could not be accurately determined; HAL doses and plasma levels were greater than with other ethnic groups, except that RHAL/HAL ratios were similar to those of the non-Chinese groups.

The stepwise regression analysis in Table 8–2 proposes that the most significant factors influencing HAL plasma concentrations were HAL dose and RHAL plasma levels. Ethnicity was only a significant factor for the Chinese and African-American groups; age and weight were not significant factors. However, these ethnic populations did not have any geriatric patients (over age 65) in this data set. Therefore, age could not be a significant factor between patients under age 65. Elderly patients were reported to require less HAL than younger patients (Vuikari et al. 1982). Weight also seemed not to a significant contributor, and other researchers have reported this finding (Forsman and Ohman 1977; Jann et al. 1985).

The relationship between RHAL and HAL plasma concentrations in Figure 8–3B appear to be nonlinear. Previous investigations have also documented a potential nonlinear relationship between HAL and RHAL concentrations (Browning et al. 1985). When HAL plasma levels were less than 10 ng/ml, no significant differences were apparent among the different ethnic populations. In general, the African-American group had the highest concentrations of RHAL plasma levels. The Hispanic group results resembled those of the African-American group, but the curve was shifted to the right. The Chinese group had lower RHAL but higher HAL plasma concentrations, as indicated by the curve shifted to the right. However, the RHAL plasma levels are disproportionally higher when HAL plasma concentrations exceed 40–50 ng/ml. Low RHAL plasma levels and high HAL concentrations have been previously reported in Chinese patients with HAL plasma levels less than 20 ng/ml (Chang et al. 1987c).

In the single-dose study of HAL and RHAL and its 4-week chronic evaluation, the metabolic rate for reduction and oxidation (the interconversion process) was similar. However, there was a wide interindividual variation in the reduction and oxidative capacities (Table 8–3). The correlation between the RHAL/HAL ratio and the interconversion clearance ($CL_{1,2}$) suggests that the ratio is only partially related to the reductive pathways. HAL and RHAL concentrations and RHAL/HAL ratios are not only related through the interconversion process but are also a function of the N-dealkylation and glucuronidation pathways. For example, patient 3 had the lowest $CL_{1,0}$ clearance, which suggests a relative deficiency in the N-dealkylation metabolism. A deficiency of this pathway could present increased HAL concentrations to the reduction route. If a low metabolic oxidation process also exists, impairment of these two pathways could result in elevated RHAL concentrations and RHAL/HAL ratios. Further, in the guinea pig model, RHAL was also reported to be glucuronidated to RHAL glucuronide and shown to undergo biliary recycling and convert back to RHAL (Eddington and Young 1990). The uridine diphosphate (UDP)–glucuronyl transferase enzyme system regulates the glucuronide metabolic pathway (Burchell et al. 1990). Differences in this enzyme complex might also exist between various individuals. Hence, interindividual and interethnic differences in RHAL/HAL ratios could be due to variabilities in these varying metabolic pathways.

The variability of the metabolic pathways could be mediated via the cytochrome P_{450} isoenzymes. The cytochrome P_{450} enzymes represent a large family of isoenzymes that mediate oxidative and reductive reactions of many drugs. The primary site of HAL conversion is in the liver, and the reduction and oxidation of HAL are most likely regulated by cytochrome P_{450} enzymes. Inaba and Kovacs (1989) reported no differences in HAL reductase activity in red blood cells between four Caucasian and four Japanese healthy volunteers; however, this small number limits the interpretation of their data. A bimodal distribution of RHAL/HAL ratios was reported in 45 Japanese patients (Someya et al. 1989). The results from that study could suggest further evidence of the interindividual variability observed within an ethnic group. Preliminary data investigating HAL disposition with polymorphic hydroxylation of debrisoquine were reported in four patients (Llerena et al. 1990). Two patients were classified as poor metabolizers, wherein the patients reported akathisia and restlessness; the HAL dosages had to be decreased in both patients. The polymorphic metabolism of HAL lends further evidence that a possible pharmacogenetic basis for HAL disposition could be involved.

The limitations of these studies are evident. In the population study, data gathered from two different countries over different time periods are subject to numerous sources of variance. Differences in prescribing patterns preclude a fixed-dose study design. The sample size for the non-Chinese groups (i.e., Caucasian, Hispanic, and African-American populations) did not equal the Chinese population. However, gathering that quantity of patients for each group could take many years. The assay methodologies differed, but the correlations between the LC and RIA for RHAL and HAL were almost equivalent. Oxidation of RHAL conversion back to HAL has not yet been quantified in non-Chinese patients. Clinical assessments for response and adverse effects were not evaluated. In the study examining the metabolic variabilities of HAL and RHAL, only a small number of patients were evaluated.

In summary, this report supports the conclusion that HAL and RHAL plasma concentrations differ among various ethnic populations, as well as among individuals within the same ethnic group. It also supports the many previous observations reported by different investigators in a smaller number of psychiatric patients. With the additional information, more advanced mathematical modeling techniques that incorporate routine plasma concentration data such as the Nonlinear Mixed Effects Model (NONMEM) can be employed to determine significant factors influencing HAL plasma concentrations (Jann et al. 1985). Understanding these complex relationships could lead to an improved usage of HAL in psychiatric patients, perhaps not only to determine therapeutic efficacy but also to outline the reasons for the lack of response in refractory patients.

REFERENCES

Altamura CA, Mauri M, Cavallaro R, et al: Reduced haloperidol/haloperidol ratio and clinical outcome in schizophrenia: preliminary evidences. Prog Neuropsychopharmacol Biol Psychiatry 12:689–694, 1988

American Psychiatric Association: Diagnostic and Statistical Manual of Mental Disorders, 3rd Edition. Washington DC, American Psychiatric Association, 1980

American Psychiatric Association: Diagnostic and Statistical Manual of Mental Disorders, 3rd Edition, Revised. Washington DC, American Psychiatric Association, 1987

Binder RL, Levy R: Extrapyramidal reactions in Asians. Am J Psychiatry 138:1243–1244, 1981

Bowen WD, Moses EL, Tolentino PJ, et al: Metabolites of haloperidol display preferential activity at sigma receptors compared to dopamine D-2 receptors. Eur J Pharmacol 177:111–118, 1990

Browning JL, Silverman PB, Harrington CA, et al: Preliminary behavioral and pharmacologic studies on the haloperidol metabolite reduced haloperidol. Society of Neuroscience Abstracts 8:470, 1982

Browning JL, Harrington CA, Davis CM: Quantification of reduced haloperidol and haloperidol by radioimmunoassay. J Immunoassay 6:45–66, 1985

Burchell B, Coughtrie MWH, Waddel L, et al: Expression and regulation of UDP-glucuronosyl-transferases. Proceedings of the Seventh International Symposium on Microsomes and Drug Oxidations (abstract), Karolinska Institute, Stockholm, Sweden, June 25–29, 1990, p 29

Chakraborty BS, Hubbard JW, Hawes EM, et al: Interconversion between haloperidol and reduced haloperidol in healthy volunteers. Eur J Clin Pharmacol 37:45–48, 1989

Chang WH, Wu HS, Tseng YT: Reduced haloperidol and haloperidol: effects on homovanillic acid in caudate and prefrontal cortex. Biol Psychiatry 22:1369–1374, 1987a

Chang WH, Chen TY, Yeh EK: Time-response curves of homovanillic acid in caudate and prefrontal cortex following acute neuroleptic administration. Psychopharmacology (Berlin) 93:403–404, 1987b

Chang WH, Chen TY, Lee CF, et al: Low plasma reduced haloperidol/haloperidol ratios in Chinese patients. Biol Psychiatry 22:1406–1408, 1987c

Chang WH, Lin SK, Jann MW, et al: Pharmacodynamics and pharmacokinetics of haloperidol and reduced haloperidol in schizophrenic patients. Biol Psychiatry 26:239–249, 1989

Cheng YF, Paalzow LK, Bondesson U, et al: Pharmacokinetics of haloperidol in psychotic patients. Psychopharmacology (Berlin) 91:410–414, 1987

Eddington ND, Young DL: Biliary excretion of reduced haloperidol glucuronide. Psychopharmacology (Berlin) 100:46–48, 1990

Ereshefsky L, Davis CM, Harrington CA, et al: Haloperidol and reduced haloperidol plasma levels in selected schizophrenic patients. J Clin Psychopharmacol 4:138–142, 1984

Forsman A, Larsson M: Metabolism of haloperidol. Current Therapeutic Research 24:567–568, 1978

Forsman A, Ohman R: Pharmacokinetic studies on haloperidol in man. Current Therapeutic Research 20:319–336, 1976

Forsman A, Ohman R: Applied pharmacokinetics of haloperidol in man. Current Therapeutic Research 21:396–410, 1977

Forsman A, Folsch G, Larsson M, et al: On the metabolism of haloperidol in man. Current Therapeutic Research 21:606–617, 1977

Froemming JH, Lam YWF, Jann MW, et al: Pharmacokinetics of haloperidol. Clin Pharmacokinet 17:396–423, 1989

Hays SE, Poland RE, Rubin RT: Prolactin releasing properties of antipsychotic and related nonantipsychotic compounds in female rats. J Pharmacol Exp Ther 214:362–367, 1980

Holley FO, Magliozzi JR, Stanski DR, et al: Haloperidol kinetics after oral and intravenous doses. Clin Pharmacol Ther 33:477–484, 1983

Inaba T, Kovacs J: Haloperidol reductase in human and guinea pig livers. Drug Metab Dispos 17:330–333, 1989

Itoh H, Yagi G, Ohtsuka N, et al: Serum level of haloperidol and its clinical significance. Prog Neuropsychopharmacol Biol Psychiatry 4:171–183, 1980

Jann MW, Ludden TM, Ereshefsky L, et al: Preliminary analysis of haloperidol population kinetics in schizophrenics. Clin Pharmacol Ther 37:203, 1985

Jann MW, Chang WH, Davis, CM, et al: Haloperidol and reduced haloperidol plasma levels in Chinese and non-Chinese psychiatric patients. Psychiatry Res 30:45–52, 1989

Jann MW, Lam YWF, Chang WH: Reversible metabolism of haloperidol and reduced haloperidol in Chinese schizophrenic patients. Psychopharmacology (Berlin) 101:107–111, 1990

Jann MW, Chang WH, Lam YWF, et al: Comparison of haloperidol and reduced haloperidol plasma levels in four different ethnic populations. Prog Neuropsychopharmacol Biol Psychiatry 16:193–202, 1992

Kalow W: Ethnic differences in drug metabolism. Clin Pharmacokinet 7:373–400, 1982

Kalow W, Otton SV, Kadar D, et al: Ethnic difference in drug metabolism: debrisoquine 4-hydroxylation in Caucasians and Orientals. Can J Physiol Pharmacol 58:1142–1144, 1980

Kirch DG, Paler MR, Egan M, et al: Electrophysiological interaction between haloperidol, reduced haloperidol, dopamine and norepinephrine and phencyclidine in rat brain. Neuropharmacol 24:375–379, 1985a

Kirch DG, Bigelow LB, Wyatt RJ: The interpretation of plasma haloperidol concentrations. Arch Gen Psychiatry 42:838–839, 1985b

Korpi ER, Phelps BH, Granger H, et al: Simultaneous determinations of haloperidol and its reduced metabolite in serum and plasma by isocratic liquid chromatography with electrochemical detection. Clin Chem 29:624–629, 1983

Korpi ER, Costakos DT, Wyatt RJ: Interconversions of haloperidol and reduced haloperidol in guinea pig and rat liver microsomes. Biochem Pharmacol 34:2923–2927, 1985a

Korpi ER, Costakos DT, Wyatt RJ: Rapid formation of reduced haloperidol in guinea pigs following haloperidol administration. Acta Pharmacol Toxicol 56:94–98, 1985b

Lam YWF, Chang WH, Jann MW, et al: Interindividual variabilities in haloperidol interconversion and the reduced haloperidol/haloperidol ratio. Neuropsychopharmacology 7:33–39, 1992

Lin KM, Finder E: Neuroleptic dosage for Asians. Am J Psychiatry 140:490–491, 1983

Lin KM, Poland RE, Lau JK, et al: Haloperidol and prolactin concentrations in Asians and Caucasians. J Clin Psychopharmacol 8:195–201, 1988

Lin KM, Poland RE, Nuccio I, et al: A longitudinal assessment of haloperidol doses and serum concentrations in Asian and Caucasian schizophrenic patients. Am J Psychiatry 146:1307–1311, 1989

Linniola M, Vuikari MM, Vaisanen K, et al: Effect of anticonvulsants on plasma haloperidol and thioridazine levels. Am J Psychiatry 137:819–821, 1980

Llerena A, Alm C, Dahl-Puustinen ML, et al: Disposition of the neuroleptics perphenazine, zuclopenthixol and haloperidol cosegregates with the polymorphic hydroxylation of debrisoquine (abstract). Proceedings of the Seventh International Symposium on Microsomes and Drug Oxidations, Karolinska Institute, Stockholm, Sweden, June 25–29, 1990, p 199

Midha KK, Chakraborty BS, Ganes DA, et al: Intersubject variation in the pharmacokinetics of haloperidol and reduced haloperidol. J Clin Psychopharmacol 9:98–104, 1989

Potkin SG, Shen Y, Pardes H, et al: Haloperidol concentrations elevated in Chinese patients. Psychiatry Res 12:167–172, 1984

Rudorfer MV, Lane EA, Chang WH, et al: Desipramine pharmacokinetics in Chinese and Caucasian volunteers. Br J Clin Pharmacol 17:433–440, 1984

Rudorfer MV, Lane EA, Potter WZ: Interethnic dissociation between debrisoquine and desipramine hydroxylation. J Clin Psychopharmacol 5:89–92, 1985

SAS Institute: SAS User's Guide: Statistics, Version 5 Edition. Cary, NC, SAS Institute, Inc, 1985

Shostak M, Perel JM, Stiller RL, et al: Plasma haloperidol and clinical response: a role for reduced haloperidol in antipsychotic activity? J Clin Psychopharmacol 7:394–400, 1987

Someya T, Takashashi S, Shibasaki M, et al: Reduced haloperidol/haloperidol ratios in plasma: polymorphism in Japanese psychiatric patients. Psychiatry Res 31:111–120, 1989

Sramek JJ, Sayles MA, Simpson GM: Neuroleptic dosage for Asians: a failure to replicate. Am J Psychiatry 143:535–536, 1986

Volavka J, Cooper TB: Review of haloperidol blood levels and clinical response: looking through the window. J Clin Psychopharmacol 7:25–30, 1987

Vuikari M, Salo H, Lamminsivu U, et al: Tolerance and serum levels of haloperidol during parental and oral haloperidol treatment in geriatric patients. Acta Psychiatr Scand 65:301–308, 1982

Yue QY, Svensson JO, Alm C, et al: Interindividual and interethnic differences in the demethylation and glucuronidation of codeine. Br J Clin Pharmacol 28:629–637, 1989

Chapter 9

Tardive Dyskinesia: Cross-Cultural Perspectives

Edmond H. Pi, M.D., Mary A. Gutierrez, Pharm.D., and Gregory E. Gray, M.D., Ph.D.

INTRODUCTION

Ethnic differences in psychopharmacology have often been noted in the medical literature. These claims include that Asians require lower doses of neuroleptics in the treatment of major psychiatric disorders (Lin and Finder 1983; Yamamoto et al. 1979) and achieve higher plasma levels of neuroleptics at the same doses than their non-Asian counterparts (Lin et al. 1989; Potkin et al. 1984). The incidence of side effects induced by neuroleptics (e.g., extrapyramidal side effects [EPS]) has been claimed to be higher among Asians than non-Asians (Binder and Levy 1981). However, these claims remain controversial (Pi et al. 1986, 1992; Sramek et al. 1986).

Tardive dyskinesia (TD), an involuntary movement disorder usually appearing late in the course of neuroleptic treatment, was described shortly after the introduction of chlorpromazine (CPZ) and other neuroleptic agents in the 1950s. The first published report of TD appeared in 1957 (Schoenecker 1957). Today, TD is a well-recognized side effect associated with the long-term use of neuroleptic therapy (Simpson et al., in press). Over the past 35 years, continuing efforts have been made to study the epidemiol-

The authors would like to give special acknowledgment to Drs. Dong-Gun Lee (Yanbian Medical College) and Zhongfu Ji and Yongzhen Weng (Hui Long Guan Hospital), People's Republic of China; Chang-Hyun Kim (National Seoul Mental Hospital) and Yong-Sik Kim (Seoul National University), Korea; Tze-Ming Leung (Lai Chi Kok Hospital), Hong Kong; Akira Kishimoto (Tottori University), Japan; and Chen-I Wu (Shantou University), People's Republic of China, for their work in the study entitled "Tardive Dyskinesia in Asians: A Multinational Study."

ogy of TD, to identify risk factors for TD, and to develop treatment modalities. However, the investigations so far have not yet led to a precise understanding of the pathophysiology of TD nor to any satisfactory treatment, though the epidemiology of TD has been better defined.

There have been many studies done on the prevalence of TD, but most have investigated Western populations. Kane and Smith (1982) reviewed 56 Western studies done between 1959 and 1979 with a combined sample size of more than 34,000 subjects. The prevalence rates in these studies ranged from 0.5% to 65%, with an average prevalence of 20%. They also found the average prevalence of spontaneous dyskinesias in patients untreated with neuroleptics to be 5%. Based on these averages, Kane and Smith estimated the prevalence of TD (corrected for spontaneous dyskinesias) to be 15%. In 1980, the American Psychiatric Association Task Force on TD similarly estimated the prevalence of TD to be 10%–20% (American Psychiatric Association 1980).

Many risk factors for the development of TD have been identified in various studies, the most consistent of which are advanced age and femaleness (Kane et al. 1986; Smith et al. 1978), although the risk associated with femaleness is much less than that for advanced age. There is a curvilinear relationship between age and TD (i.e., the risk remains stable between the ages of 20 and 40, then rises sharply with age; Kane et al. 1986). Also, advanced age is more likely to be associated with persistent TD (Kane et al. 1986). Other possible risk factors for TD include affective disorders, early onset of EPS, presence of severe EPS that cannot be suppressed by antiparkinsonian medication, and duration of neuroleptic treatment (Chouinard et al. 1986; Kane et al. 1986). Despite numerous epidemiologic studies of TD, few have focused on the role of ethnicity as a risk factor.

In this chapter, we present a review of five epidemiologic studies dealing with TD in Asian psychiatric patients that were published in English-language publications. The studies had sample sizes ranging from 115 to 982, with a total of 3,006 subjects. The emphasis will be placed on cross-cultural aspects of TD, investigating the relationship of TD with demographic, ethnic, clinical, and drug history variables. Clinical implications and recommendations for future studies are discussed.

REVIEW OF CROSS-CULTURAL STUDIES IN ASIAN PSYCHIATRIC PATIENTS

There is limited evidence that there may be differences in the prevalence of TD among various ethnic groups: Chinese in China (Ko et al. 1989; Pi et al. 1990) and Hong Kong (Chiu et al. 1992); Asians in America (Pi et al. 1992); Japanese in Japan (Binder et al. 1987; Pi et al. 1990); and Koreans in Korea and China (Pi et al. 1990). These studies are summarized in Table 9–1.

Binder and colleagues (1987) studied 126 inpatients in Tokyo and Osaka, Japan. They found a point prevalence of TD of 20.6%, which is consistent with Western studies (Kane and Smith 1982; Smith et al. 1978). The authors stated that the recommended doses of neuroleptics were relatively low in Japan when compared to Western recommendations, but that polypharmacy was common in Japan (stemming from the tradition of Asian herb medicine in which the "best" prescriptions usually included a mixture of many ingredients). The actual mean total daily dose for the combination of neuroleptic agents given to the inpatients in this study was 1,634 mg CPZ equivalents, hardly a low dose. In this study, the risk factors for TD that were identified were advanced age and duration of neuroleptic treatment (as measured by the length of hospitalization). Duration was only associated with moderate to severe TD, not with mild TD. This study was limited by the inclusion of neuroleptics available in Japan but not in the United States.

The prevalence of TD in 866 Chinese chronic schizophrenic patients in a psychiatric hospital in Shanghai was studied by Ko and colleagues (1989). The point prevalence in this study was 8.4%—less than the usual prevalence in Western studies. The authors attribute this low prevalence rate to low neuroleptic doses, averaging only 311 ± 254 mg CPZ equivalents (mean ± SD). The authors also stated that Chinese physicians historically prescribed relatively low doses of neuroleptics. (There are studies indicating that the point prevalence of TD is lower in countries where smaller doses of neuroleptics have historically been used [Smith and Baldessarini 1980; Yassa et al. 1984].) Risk factors identified in this study were advanced age, high daily neuroleptic dose, long duration of treatment, family history of

Table 9–1. Summary of epidemiologic studies of tardive dyskinesia in Asians

Study	Site(s)	*N*	% Female	Average age	% Schizophrenia	TD Prevalence			Average neuroleptic dose (CPZ equiv.)	% taking antiparkinsonian drugs	Risk factors
						Mild	Moderate to severe	Total			
Binder et al. 1987	Japan	126	48%	38	94%	6.4%	14.2%	20.6%	1,634	100%	Older age Increased length of hospitalization
Ko et al. 1989	China	866	26%	43	100%			8.4%	311	N/A	Older age High neuroleptic dose Long duration of neuroleptic use History of EPS Family history of schizophrenia
Pi et al. 1990	China, Hong Kong, Japan, Korea	982	42%	44	91%	11.2%	5.8%	17.0%	546	58%	Older age Low neuroleptic dose Treatment in a site other than Beijing
Pi et al. 1991	Los Angeles, CA (mixed Asianethnicity)	115	51%	38	63%	9.6%	6.1%	15.7%	300	65%	Older age Low neuroleptic dose
Chiu et al. 1992	Hong Kong	917	45%	46	66%			9.3%	896	71%	Older age Low neuroleptic dose

Note. CPZ = chlorpromazine; TD = tardive dyskinesia; EPS = extrapyramidal side effects.

schizophrenia, and a history of acute EPS.

The prevalence of TD was studied in 115 Asian-American outpatients (Pi et al. 1992). The ethnic composition of the subject group was 35.7% Chinese (*n* = 41), 23.5% Korean (*n* = 27), 20.9% Japanese (*n* = 24), 17.4% Pilipino (*n* = 20), 1.7% Vietnamese (*n* = 2), and 0.9% Cambodian (*n* = 1). The results showed moderate TD in 6.1% (*n* = 7) of the patients, mild TD in 9.6% (*n* = 11), and no severe TD. The total prevalence in this study population was 15.7% (*n* = 18). Age was the only significant risk factor for TD that was identified. Subjects aged 40 to 49 were 3 times more likely to have TD than those under age 40, and subjects over age 50 were roughly 8 times more likely to have TD than those under age 40.

Chiu and colleagues (1992) studied 917 Chinese patients in Hong Kong. The point prevalence of TD in this study was 9.3% (*n* = 85). Of these patients, 84.7% (*n* = 72) had persistent TD. The majority of patients (*n* = 602) had a diagnosis of schizophrenia; among them, the prevalence of TD was 8.5% (*n* = 51). The risk factors identified in this study are advanced age and lower current dose of neuroleptic.

A multinational study of TD in Asians was also carried out (Pi et al. 1990). The subjects were 18 years of age or older, of either sex, and currently receiving psychiatric inpatient treatment; all had a history of at least 3 months of neuroleptic use. Nine hundred and eighty-two hospitalized psychiatric patients from Beijing (*n* = 232) and Yanji (*n* = 291), China; Hong Kong (*n* = 155); Seoul, Korea (*n* = 165); and Tottori, Japan (*n* = 139), were examined for abnormal movements using the Abnormal Involuntary Movement Scale (AIMS; National Institute of Mental Health [NIMH] 1975). Each patient was evaluated by the senior investigator as well as psychiatrists at each hospital. Schooler and Kane's (1982) Research Diagnostic Criteria (RDC) for TD were used to establish the diagnosis. Other demographic and clinical data were obtained from the patients' charts (see Table 9–2). There were no patients who had any identified neurologic condition that could cause a movement disorder, such as Wilson's disease or Huntington's chorea.

The overall prevalence of TD was 17% (*n* = 167; 11.2% mild *n* = 110, 4.8% moderate *n* = 47, and 1.0% severe *n* = 10), which is

Table 9–2. Description of subjects in a study by Pi et al. (1990)

Site	*N*	% Female	Average age	% Schizophrenia	Average duration of illness (years)	Average neuroleptic dose (CPZ equivalent)	% Taking antiparkinsonian drugs
Beijing, China	232	49	42	95	18	580	74
Yanji, China							
Ethnic Chinese	70	23	40	97	16	354	36
Ethnic Koreans	221	39	43	88	17	283	37
Hong Kong	115	51	53	94	23	455	44
Seoul, Korea	165	53	35	82	10	1,051	63
Tottori, Japan	139	38	51	91	24	1,131	96

Note. CPZ = chlorpromazine.

very similar to previous studies in a variety of different Western patient populations. However, the 232 subjects from Beijing, China, showed a prevalence rate of only 8.2%, similar to the two studies conducted in Hong Kong (Chiu et al. 1992) and Shanghai (Ko et al. 1989). The prevalence of TD was 15.8% (n = 26) for the Koreans in Seoul, Korea; 20.4% (n = 45) for the Koreans in Yanji, China; 19.1% (n = 22) for the Chinese in Hong Kong; and 18.6% (n = 13) for the Chinese in Yanji, China (see Figure 9–1). Average current neuroleptic doses in CPZ equivalents ranged from 283 mg in Yanji, China, to 1,131 mg in Tottori, Japan (see Table 9–2).

Because of significant confounding effects, multiple logistic regression analysis was used to estimate the effects of a given risk factor while controlling for all other risk factors. Using this approach, the significant risk factors identified were age 50+ years (odds ratio [OR] = 2.8), current neuroleptic dose < 200 mg CPZ equivalents (OR = 1.9), and site, with patients outside Beijing

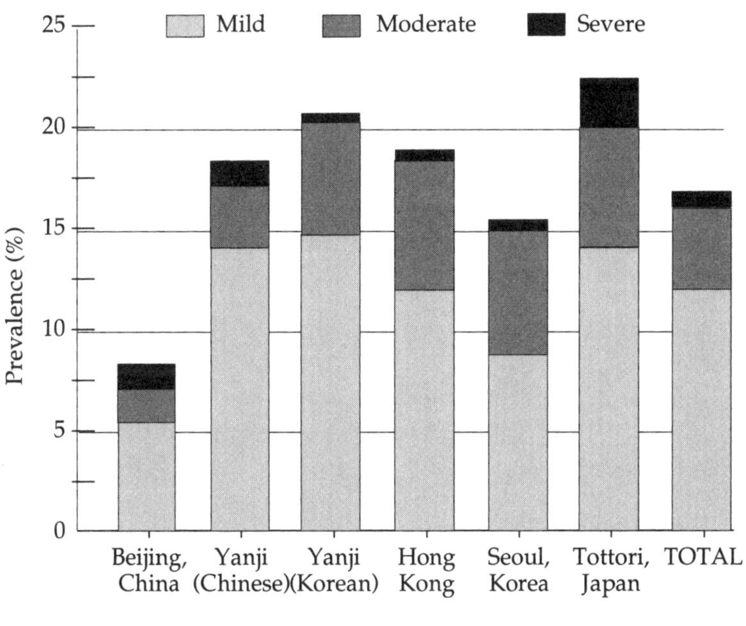

Figure 9–1. Prevalence of tardive dyskinesia in six study samples. Adapted from Pi et al. 1990.

having a risk 1.9 to 2.9 times greater than those in Beijing (see Table 9–3).

These findings confirm that the risk of TD increases with age, as has been demonstrated in other studies. There was a significant difference in TD prevalence among different sites with the same ethnic group (e.g., the Koreans in Korea and China differed by 4.5%, and the Chinese in Hong Kong and Yanji differed from those in Beijing by 11.2% and 10.4%, respectively). Reasons for such differences are unclear. Similarity in prevalence among the Chinese and Korean patients in Yanji, China, suggests that differences are more apt to be due to environmental factors than genetics. The differences in TD prevalence among the sites were not secondary to differences in age between the study groups, although the higher prevalence in Korea and Japan may be a reflection of higher average neuroleptic dosages. Duration of illness was not an independent risk factor after controlling for age. The third factor identified was lower current neuroleptic dose. Risk of TD was greatest in patients on the lowest current neuroleptic dosage in this study (see Table 9–3). This may reflect the lowering of doses after TD develops. Lower doses of neuroleptics may also have an unmasking effect for the movement disorder. We con-

Table 9–3. Risk factors for tardive dyskinesia derived from logistic regression analysis of data from a study by Pi et al. (1990)

Risk factor	Odds ratio	*P*
Age (years)		
< 30	1.00	
30–49	1.55	NS
50+	2.79	.0035
Daily neuroleptic dose (CPZ equivalent)		
< 200	1.86	.0037
200+	1.00	
Site/ethnicity		
Beijing	1.00	
Yanji (Chinese)	2.58	.0194
Yanji (Korean)	2.95	.0009
Hong Kong	1.94	.0465
Seoul	2.72	.0029
Tottori	2.89	.0011

Note. CPZ = chlorpromazine.

cluded that environmental factors (e.g., prescribing practices) at a given site were more likely to explain differences between sites than genetics or ethnicity.

DISCUSSION

Methodological Problems of TD Studies

There are significant difficulties conducting studies comparing cross-cultural differences in psychopharmacology. The difficulties include limited sample sizes, mixed ethnic groups, unavailability of drug histories for each patient, variable diagnostic criteria for both psychiatric disorders and TD, different examination techniques, and uncertain interrater reliability among research groups.

The AIMS was developed by NIMH for use in evaluating the presence and severity of movements consistent with TD (NIMH 1975). Although originally developed for research purposes, the AIMS is now the most widely used test for TD in clinical practice. However this test was not available until 1975; therefore, studies before 1975 were conducted with different criteria for TD. The 56 studies reviewed by Kane and colleagues (1986) were done between 1959 and 1979, implying that most of these studies did not use the AIMS for evaluation. The 20% prevalence rate from these studies may be somewhat biased by the criteria the studies used. However, even with the AIMS, investigators can use different criteria for the diagnosis of TD. All five studies we present used the AIMS, but there was no consistent scoring criteria for defining TD. In three of the studies (Chiu et al. 1992; Pi et al. 1990, 1992) used a score of 2 or more in at least two body parts as indicating mild TD. Ko and colleagues (1989) used a global score of 2 or greater for the presence of TD. Binder and colleagues (1987) used a score of 2 or more in at least one body part as the diagnosis. Therefore, the wide range of prevalence rates (8%–21%) may be a reflection of the three sets of criteria used for the diagnosis of TD.

Another issue is interrater reliability among research groups. The AIMS is scored by rating severity of movements in seven specific body parts and by making global ratings of severity of movements, incapacitation, and subjective awareness and distress of the patient. Each rating is given a score from 0 to 4, with 0 as none, 1 as minimal or extreme normal, 2 as mild, 3 as moderate, and 4 as severe. The AIMS developed by the NIMH has no specific instructions on how to score movements. Subjective interrater differences are inevitable and can contribute to the differences in TD prevalence reported by different investigators. Also, the original AIMS has a notation that movements seen only upon activation should be rated 1 point less than the severity observed. Several investigators have reported that they do not follow these instructions (Lane et al. 1985; Munetz and Benjamin 1988; Smith et al. 1978). They believe that there is no evidence that a movement occurring only upon activation has less significance than a movement occurring spontaneously. In addition, they believe that the activating procedures resemble movements that the patient makes in the course of normal daily activities. Therefore, these raters will score the patients' AIMS higher than those following the original instructions.

Age and Gender

The increased risk of TD with advanced age has been well established in the literature, and all the studies reviewed here confirm this association. To date, age is the only unequivocal risk factor in TD.

Surprisingly, none of these studies found the significant association between femaleness and TD that has been reported in American, Canadian, and French studies (Kane and Smith 1982; Yesavage et al. 1982). The reason for such a discrepancy is unclear but may reflect a confounding of femaleness with other risk factors such as age or neuroleptic dose. Kane and colleagues (1986) found femaleness to be a risk factor even after stratifying by age. However, one study (Pi et al. 1990) controlled for age using multiple logistic regression and failed to identify femaleness as a risk factor.

Neuroleptic Dose and Duration of Neuroleptic Treatment

Although a low dose of neuroleptic for Asian patients is commonly recommended in clinical practice and in the literature, the current mean total daily neuroleptic dose prescribed in these studies was similar to, if not higher than, usual doses in Western countries.

The use of relatively low doses of neuroleptics was proposed as a possible explanation for the low prevalence rate of TD reported in one study (Ko et al. 1989). On the other hand, an interesting inverse relation between the presence of TD and current neuroleptic dosages was found in four studies, with the patients with TD receiving lower current doses of neuroleptics than patients without TD (Chiu et al. 1992; Pi et al. 1990, 1992; Sramek et al. 1991). This may be explained by the concept of "covert" TD (i.e., higher doses of neuroleptics are more likely to suppress TD movements). Also, this may suggest that the treating physicians reduced the doses of neuroleptics following the detection of TD symptoms in patients. This is a limitation of the cross-sectional study design in which current dosages are associated with TD rather than past dosages. Such discrepancies between studies may also be attributed to the lack of reliable information of drug history on patients and to the researchers' arbitrary definition of "daily neuroleptic dose" based on retrospective chart review, which provides only limited information.

A positive association between duration of neuroleptic treatment and prevalence of TD was found in two studies (Ko et al. 1989; Pi et al. 1990). As pointed out by Muscettola and colleagues (1989), who conducted a TD prevalence study in Italy and made the same finding, this might be partly attributed to confounding effect of age. This was indeed the case in one study (Pi et al. 1990) in which duration of treatment was no longer a significant risk factor after controlling for age. Although the development of TD may be related to cumulative neuroleptic exposure as found by Kane and colleagues (1986), in this kind of cross-sectional study, it is generally impossible to calculate the cumulative neuroleptic exposure before the onset of TD in the patients. It is therefore difficult to conclude that cumulative neuroleptic exposure is an independent risk factor for the development of TD. Using CPZ equivalents as the standard for various neuroleptic exposure or for current daily dose is also subject to error, because tables of CPZ equivalents are only available for neuroleptics released in the United States. For example, one study in Japan (Binder et al. 1987) as well as part of another study (Pi et al. 1990) conducted in Japan involved Japanese neuroleptics not available in the United States and for which there is no established method for conversion to CPZ equivalents. The conversion in these studies was based on the *Japanese Drug Directory* (Japanese Pharmaceutical Trading Association 1987).

Prevalence of TD and Ethnicity

Giving that age, sex, and exposure to neuroleptics are considered to be the only consistent risk factors for the development of TD, theoretically there should be no differences in the prevalence of TD among different ethnic populations. Two studies (Binder et al. 1987; Pi et al. 1990) reported no significant difference of TD prevalence between Asian and non-Asian patients. This raises a challenge to the common belief that Asians are more sensitive to both therapeutic effects and side effects of neuroleptics. Such a lack of difference in the prevalence of TD is also reported in other cross-cultural studies involving non-Asian populations. For example, Muscettola and colleagues (1989) reported a 19% TD prevalence ($n = 315$) among 1,651 psychiatric inpatients and outpatients in Italy. Sramek and colleagues (1991) reported no difference in TD prevalence among 491 Caucasian, black, and Hispanic hospitalized psychiatric patients; the average TD prevalence for the whole group was 17.7% ($n = 87$). Difference in TD prevalence among different sites with the same ethnic groups (Ko et al. 1989; Pi et al. 1990), coupled with similarity in prevalence among different ethnic groups (Binder et al. 1987; Kane and Smith 1982; Pi et al. 1990; Sramek et al. 1986), suggests that differences are more apt to be due to environmental factors than to genetics.

Severity of TD

Most cases of TD appear to be mild or moderate, with severe TD occurring rarely. No cases of severe TD were found in one study (Pi et al. 1992), which concurs with previously published data on Hungarian schizophrenic patients (Gardos et al. 1980). This suggests that cases of severe TD are relatively rare and are not likely to be detected in studies with relatively small sample sizes.

CONCLUSION

After reviewing the epidemiologic data on Asian populations with TD, several points are worth noting. First, it is difficult to compare results between studies because of differences in research designs. Nevertheless, there are several consistent findings. The only consistent risk factor is age; being female is not a consistent risk factor. Other possible risk factors mentioned include duration of treatment, length of hospitalization, duration of psychiatric disorder, family history of schizophrenia, and history of acute EPS. Current daily dose of neuroleptics is inversely related to TD in cross-sectional studies; this may be an artifact of study design. There is currently little convincing evidence that differences in the prevalence of TD truly exist between Asians and non-Asians.

To assess the degree of neuroleptic usage as a risk factor for the development of TD, cohort studies in which the dosage and duration of neuroleptic use are accurately determined must be conducted. One hopes that certain neurobiological measurements such as receptor sensitivity can be identified and used to differentiate genetically determined individual susceptibility of developing TD from environmentally determined factors (e.g., physicians' prescribing habits). This can only be achieved through a cohort study in which dosage information and the incidence rate of TD can be accurately assessed. Such a study is now potentially feasible, because large numbers of patients of Asian ancestry reside in several metropolitan areas in North America and because of increasing collaboration among researchers in Pacific Rim countries.

Meanwhile, as there is no safe and effective treatment for TD, prevention is the major aim regardless of a patient's culture. This goal can be best achieved by prescribing neuroleptics only when clinically indicated, prescribing the lowest effective dose of neuroleptics for any psychiatric patient with or without symptoms of TD, evaluating the patient periodically for unusual movements, and reviewing indications for continuing neuroleptic therapy.

REFERENCES

American Psychiatric Association: Tardive dyskinesia: summary of a Task Force Report of the American Psychiatric Association. Am J Psychiatry 137:1163–1172, 1980

Binder RL, Levy R: Extrapyramidal reactions in Asians. Am J Psychiatry 138:1243–1244, 1981

Binder RL, Kazamatsuri H, Nishimura T, et al: Tardive dyskinesia and neuroleptic-induced parkinsonism in Japan. Am J Psychiatry 144:1494–1496, 1987

Chiu H, Shum P, Lau J, et al: Prevalence of tardive dyskinesia, tardive dystonia and respiratory dyskinesia in Chinese psychiatric patients in Hong Kong. Am J Psychiatry 149:1081–1085, 1992

Chouinard G, Annable L, Mercier P, et al: A five-year follow-up study of tardive dyskinesia. Psychopharmacol Bull 22:259–263, 1986

Gardos G, Samu I, Kallos M, et al: Absence of severe tardive dyskinesia in Hungarian schizophrenic outpatients. Psychopharmacology (Berlin) 71:29–34, 1980

Japanese Pharmaceutical Trading Association: Japanese Drug Directory, 3rd Edition. Tokyo, Japan, Japanese Pharmaceutical Trading Association, 1987

Kane JM, Smith JM: Tardive dyskinesia: prevalence and risk factors, 1959 to 1979. Arch Gen Psychiatry 39:473–481, 1982

Kane JM, Woerner M, Borenstein M, et al: Integrating incidence and prevalence of tardive dyskinesia. Psychopharmacol Bull 22:254–258, 1986

Ko GN, Zhang LD, Yan WW, et al: The Shanghai 800: prevalence of tardive dyskinesia in a Chinese psychiatric hospital. Am J Psychiatry 146:387–389, 1989

Lane RD, Glazer WH, Hansen TE, et al: Assessment of tardive dyskinesia using the Abnormal Involuntary Movement Scale. J Nerv Ment Dis 173:353–357, 1985

Lin KM, Finder EJ: Neuroleptic dosage in Asians. Am J Psychiatry 140:490–491, 1983

Lin KM, Poland RE, Nuccio I, et al: A longitudinal assessment of haloperidol doses and serum concentrations in Asian and Caucasian schizophrenic patients. Am J Psychiatry 146:1307–1311, 1989

Munetz MR, Benjamin S: How to examine patients using the Abnormal Involuntary Movement Scale. Hosp Community Psychiatry 39:1172–1177, 1988

Muscettola G, Pampallona S, Barbato G, et al: Tardive dyskinesia in Italy: preliminary findings. Arch Gen Psychiatry 46:754–755, 1989

National Institute of Mental Health: Early clinical drug evaluation unit: Abnormal Involuntary Movement Scale (AIMS). Intercom 4:3–6, 1975
Pi EH, Jain A, Simpson GM: Review and survey of different prescribing practice in Asia, in Biological Psychiatry 1985. Edited by Shagaas C, et al. New York, Elsevier, 1986, pp 1536–1538
Pi EH, Gray GE, Lee DG, et al: Tardive dyskinesia in Asians: a multinational study. Paper presented at the annual meeting of the American Psychiatric Association, New York, May 1990
Pi EH, Kusuda M, Gray GE, et al: Cross-cultural psychopharmacology: neuroleptic-induced movements disorders, in Phenothiazines and Structurally Related Compounds. Edited by Keyzer H, Eckert GM, Forrest IS, et al. Melbourne, FL, Krieger Publishing, 1992, pp 399–408
Potkin SG, Shen Y, Pardes H, et al: Haloperidol concentrations elevated in Chinese patients. Psychiatric Res 12:167–172, 1984
Schoenecker M: Ein eigentumliches Syndrom im oralen Bereich bei Megaphenapplikation. Nervenarzt 28:35, 1957
Schooler NR, Kane JM: Research diagnoses for tardive dyskinesia. Arch Gen Psychiatry 39:486–487, 1982
Simpson GM, Pi EH, Sramek JJ: Neuroleptics and antipsychotic drugs, in Meyler's Side Effects of Drugs, 12th Edition. Edited by Dukes MNG. Amsterdam, Netherlands, Excerpta Medica Tertiary Publications (in press)
Smith JM, Baldessarini RJ: Changes in prevalence, severity and recovery in tardive dyskinesia with age. Arch Gen Psychiatry 37:1368–1373, 1980
Smith JM, Oswald WT, Kucharski LT, et al: Tardive dyskinesia: age and sex differences in hospitalized schizophrenics. Psychopharmacology (Berlin) 58:207–211, 1978
Sramek JJ, Sayles MA, Simpson GM: Neuroleptic dosage for Asians: a failure to replicate. Am J Psychiatry 143:535–536, 1986
Sramek JJ, Roy S, Ahrens T, et al: Prevalence of tardive dyskinesia among three ethnic groups of chronic psychiatric patients. Hosp Community Psychiatry 42:590–592, 1991
Yamamoto J, Fung D, Lo S, et al: Psychopharmacology for Asian Americans and Pacific Islanders. Psychopharmacol Bull 15:29–31, 1979
Yassa R, Nair V, Schwartz G: Tardive dyskinesia and the primary psychiatric diagnosis. Psychosomatics 25:135–138, 1984
Yesavage JA, Bourgeois M, Kraemer H, et al: Prevalence of tardive dyskinesia in 3,140 French inpatients. J Nerv Ment Dis 170:111–112, 1982

Chapter 10

Genetic Polymorphisms of Alcohol-Metabolizing Enzymes Related to Alcohol Sensitivity and Alcoholic Diseases

Akira Yoshida, Ph.D.

A higher frequency of alcohol sensitivity among Asians than in Caucasians has been recognized for a long time. Wolff (1972, 1973) presented the first systematic study of the racial difference in alcohol sensitivity using adults and young children who were not preexposed to alcohol. He observed that more than 80% of Asians and about 50% of American Indians were alcohol sensitive ("alcohol flusher" subjects), whereas less than 10% of Caucasians exhibited alcohol flushing. Wolff concluded that the difference is a genetic—not acquired—characteristic.

Ingested ethanol is oxidized by alcohol dehydrogenase (ADH) to acetaldehyde, and subsequently further oxidized by aldehyde dehydrogenase (ALDH) to produce nontoxic acetate. Blood acetaldehyde level, but not alcohol level, is substantially higher in alcohol-sensitive Asians than in nonsensitive individuals (Mizoi et al. 1979). Alcohol sensitivity among Asians has now been proven to be due to the genetic differences of alcohol-metabolizing enzymes.

ALCOHOL DEHYDROGENASE

ADH isozymes of humans and other mammals are grouped in distinctive "classes" based on their enzymatic characteristics and

---

This work was supported by U.S. Public Health Service Grant # AA05763.

structural similarities (Table 10–1, ref. in Yoshida et al. 1991). The class I ADHs exhibit a high activity for ethanol oxidation and play a major role in ethanol oxidation. The class I enzymes also oxidize neurotransmitters. They are most abundant in the liver and exist also in other tissues, including the lungs and kidneys, but are not detectable in the brain, skin fibroblasts, and red blood cells. The class II ADH is primarily found in the liver. A similar but not identical class II ADH exists in the stomach (Moreno and Parés 1991; Yin et al. 1990). It is known that females are more susceptible to alcoholic liver injury than are males. It was reported that a significant amount of orally ingested ethanol was metabolized in the stomach of males, but not of females, and ADH activity of stomach mucous membranes is substantially higher in males than in females (Frezza et al. 1990). Our research

Table 10–1. ADH genes and polymorphisms

ADH class	Locus	Common alleles	Subunit	Mutation site	Gene frequencies
I	ADH_1	ADH_1	α		~100%
	ADH_2	ADH_2^1	β_1		Wild type, > 90% in Caucasians
	ADH_2	ADH_2^2	β_2	Arg→His at position 47	Common in Asians (~70%)
		ADH_2^3	β_3	Arg→Cys at position 369	Common in blacks (~16%)
	ADH_3	ADH_3^1	γ_1		Wild type, > 90% in Asians
		ADH_3^2	γ_2	Arg→Glu at position 271 Ile→Val at position 349	Common in Caucasians (~40%)
II	ADH_4	ADH_4^1	π_1		
		ADH_4^2	π_2	Arg→Lys at position 302 Val→Ile at position 312	
III	ADH_5	ADH_5	χ		
	ADH_6	ADH_6			

Note. Arg = arginine; His = histidine; Cys = cysteine; Glu = glutamine; Ile = isoleucine; Val = valine; Lys = lysine.
Source. Data from Yoshida et al. 1991.

team cloned and characterized the ADH_6 gene, and we found that the gene is expressed in the stomach and has a hormone-responsive element (Yasunami et al. 1991). The enzyme produced by the ADH_6 gene exhibited class II ADH characteristics. The ADH_6 gene could be responsible for the sex-dependent ADH isozyme. The class III ADH is found in all tissues examined, including the brain, testes, and red blood cells. All ADH genes are located on chromosome 4q21-25 in humans.

The ADH_2 (for β subunit), ADH_3 (for γ subunit), and ADH_4 (for π subunit) are polymorphic (i.e., there is more than one common allele in these loci). The frequency of the wild type (usual) ADH_2^1 gene exceeds 90% in Caucasians, but it is only about 30% in Asians. Instead, the atypical ADH_2^2 gene is more common (70%) in Asians. Another atypical gene, ADH_2^3, is fairly common in blacks (Table 10–1).

Two common genes, the wild type ADH_3^1 gene and variant ADH_2^3, are found in Caucasians, whereas the frequency of the variant gene is low in Asians.

The genomic difference between the wild type ADH_2^1 gene and the atypical Asian type ADH_2^2 gene is G/C→A/T base transition in exon 3, which results in a single amino acid substitution, Arg→His at the 47th position of the enzyme. The molecular difference between the wild type β_1 and the variant β_3 is Arg→Cys at the 369th position generated by C/G→T/A base transition in exon 9. The specific activities of the atypical $\beta_2\beta_2$ and $\beta_3\beta_3$ enzymes are more than two orders of magnitude higher than the usual $\beta_1\beta_1$ enzyme at the physiological pH. The β subunit is more abundant than other subunits in the liver, and therefore the isozymes consisting of β subunit are considered to play a major role in ethanol oxidation. Although the atypical isozymes have much higher specific activity than the usual enzyme, the rate of ethanol elimination in subjects with the atypical enzyme is not much different from that in other subjects. This is because ADH action is reversible and affected by nicotinamide adenine dinucleotide/reduced nicotinamide adenine dinucleotide (NAD/NADH) ratio and concentrations of acetaldehyde and other metabolites in the tissues.

Two amino acid substitutions (i.e., Arg→Glu at position 271 and Ile→Val at position 349) are found in the common γ_2 enzyme.

The normal $\gamma_1\gamma_1$ enzyme is about 2 times more active than the variant $\gamma_2\gamma_2$ enzyme.

ALDEHYDE DEHYDROGENASE

Several ALDH isozymes have been distinguished based on the separation by physicochemical methods, tissue and subcellular distributions, and enzymatic properties (Table 10–2; ref. in Yoshida et al. 1991). The cytosolic liver $ALDH_1$ and the mitochondrial liver $ALDH_2$, which exhibit high activities for the oxidation of acetaldehyde, are considered to play a major role in acetaldehyde detoxification in the liver. Approximately 50% of Asians lack $ALDH_2$ activity in their livers (Figure 10–1). The deficiency is due to the genomic mutation in the $ALDH_2$ locus (i.e., a point mutation G/C→A/T in exon 12), which results in Glu→Lys substitution at position 487 (Yoshida et al. 1984; Hsu et al. 1985). The frequency of the variant $ALDH_2^2$ gene is about 30% in Japanese and null (or very low) in Caucasians (Shibuya and Yoshida 1988a). The heterozygous $ALDH_2^1/ALDH_2^2$ as well as homozygous atypical $ALDH_2^2/ALDH_2^2$ lack $ALDH_2$ activity in their livers (i.e., the variant $ALDH_2^2$ gene is dominant in the expression of enzyme activity; Table 10–3).

In contrast to the $ALDH_2$, common $ALDH_1$ variants have not been found. A variant with severely diminished catalytic activity was found in about 5% of Japanese (Yoshida 1983), and a variant associated with different electrophoretic mobility was found in two Asian subjects (Eckey et al. 1986). Two $ALDH_1$ variants with diminished activity were found in Caucasian subjects who exhibited alcohol flushing (Yoshida et al. 1989).

Based on the multiplicity of $ALDH_3$ isozymes in stomach samples, the existence of two nonallelic genes ($ALDH_{3a}$ and $ALDH_{3b}$) was proposed in humans (Yin et al. 1988). However, our research team recently cloned the $ALDH_3$ gene and demonstrated that the single gene is responsible for the formation of $ALDH_3$ isozymes (Hsu et al. 1992). The $ALDH_3$ isozymes either cannot be detected or are expressed at low levels in normal liver tissue, but at high levels in the stomach and hepatoma cells and presumably also in other carcinoma tissues. The $ALDH_3$ locus is probably polymorphic in certain populations (Duley et al. 1985; Hopkinson et al.

Table 10–2. Human ALDH isozymes

Isozyme	Major tissues	Subcellular localization	Major Substrate, Km (μM) and pH	Subunit MW	Subunit/active enzyme
$ALDH_1$	Liver	C	Acetaldehyde, 22 μM at pH 7.5	54,000	4
$ALDH_2$	Liver	M	Acetaldehyde, 3.5 μM at pH 7.5	54,000	4
$ALDH_3$	Liver, stomach	C	Heptaldehyde, 11 μM at pH 8.5	54,000	2
$ALDH_4$	Liver	M	Glutamic-γ-semialdehyde, 100 μ at pH 7.0	70,600	2
γ-ABDH major minor	Liver	N	γ-aminobutyraldehyde, 13.8 μM at pH 7.4 8.0 μM at pH 7.4	54,000	4
$ALDH_x$	Liver, testis	M	Unknown	54,000	Unknown
$ALDH_{2a}$ (disulfiram sensitive)	Brain	M	Acetaldehyde, 1 μM at pH 9.0 dopaldehyde, 1 μM at pH 9.0	54,000	4
$ALDH_{2b}$ (disulfiram insensitive)	Brain	M	Acetaldehyde, 1 μM at pH 9.0 dopaldehyde, 0.5 μM at pH 9.0	54,000	4
Saliva ALDH	Saliva	C	Acetaldehyde, 106 μM at pH 8.0	48,000	4

Note. ALDH = aldehyde dehydrogenase.

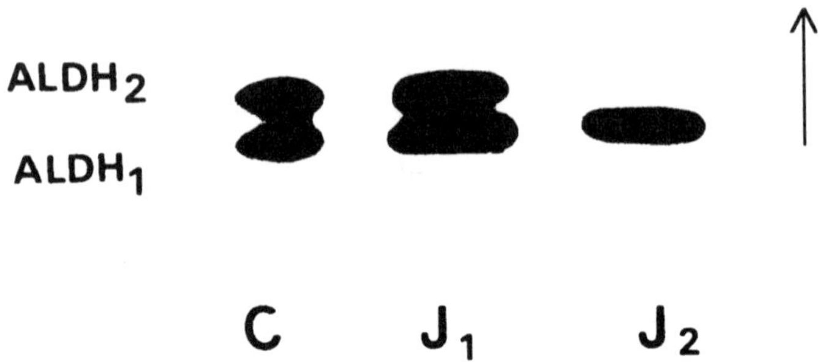

Figure 10–1. Starch gel electrophoretic patterns of human liver aldehyde dehydrogenase (ALDH) isozymes. C = usual pattern for Caucasian liver; J_1 = usual pattern for Japanese liver; J_2 = atypical pattern for Japanese liver lacking mitochondrial $ALDH_2$.

Table 10–3. Phenotypes and genotypes of $ALDH_2$

Sample code	$ALDH_2$ isozyme	Genotypes
87-33	+	1-1
88-52	+	1-1
A85-31	–	1-2
88-42	–	2-2
88-54	–	1-2
88-36	–	1-2
87-17	–	2-2
A85-33	+	1-1
88-8	+	1-1
A84-48	–	1-2
A87-35	–	2-2
A88-55	–	1-2

Note. ALDH = aldehyde dehydrogenase; + = usual phenotype with $ALDH_2$ band; – = atypical phenotype lacking $ALDH_2$ band.
Source. Data from Yoshida et al. 1990.

1985). The newly discovered $ALDH_x$ gene, which is expressed in testes, is polymorphic (Hsu and Chang 1991). Differences of enzymatic properties of normal and variant-type enzymes produced by these two $ALDH_x$ genes have not yet been elucidated.

GENETIC BACKGROUND FOR ALCOHOL SENSITIVITY AND ALCOHOLIC DISEASES

Since the genomic structures of ADH and ALDH loci and the genomic abnormalities of the common variant genes were elucidated, it has become possible to determine the genotypes of these loci by hybridization of DNA fragments with a pair of allele-specific oligonucleotide probes (Hsu et al. 1987; Ikuta et al. 1988).

The genotypes of the ADH_2 and $ALDH_2$ loci of Japanese subjects who exhibited alcohol flushing or nonflushing, patients with alcoholic liver diseases, and control subjects have been determined by our research group (Shibuya and Yoshida 1988a, 1988b; Shibuya et al. 1989). These findings have been subsequently replicated by other investigators who have also extended the study to other Asian populations (Harada 1990; Singh et al. 1989; Thomasson et al. 1991).

The most remarkable genomic difference between alcohol-flushing subjects and nonflushing subjects and between alcoholic patients and control subjects is the frequencies of the wild type $ALDH_2^1$ and the atypical Asian type $ALDH_2^2$ genes (Table 10–4 and Figure 10–2). Virtually all Japanese subjects who exhibit alcohol flushing are either heterozygous type 1/2 or homozygous atypical type 2/2 at the $ALDH_2$ locus; conversely, most pa-

Table 10–4. Genotypes of $ALDH_2$ locus in Japanese subjects

	Genotypes			**Gene frequency**	
	1-1	**1-2**	**2-2**	**$ALDH_2^1$**	**$ALDH_2^2$**
Control subjects ($n = 49$)	21	22	6	0.65	0.35
Patients with alcoholic liver disease ($n = 23$)	20	3	0	0.93	0.07
Alcohol flusher subjects ($n = 22$)	1	14	7	0.36	0.64
Nonflusher subjects ($n = 8$)	7	1	0	0.94	0.06

tients with alcoholic liver diseases are homozygous usual type 1/1. One can conclude that Japanese with genotypes $ALDH_2^1$/ $ALDH_2^2$ or $ALDH_2^2$ /$ALDH_2^2$ are alcohol sensitive, cannot drink a large amount of alcohol, and do not have a strong alcohol-seeking tendency. Consequently, they are at low risk for developing alcoholic liver diseases. Harada (1990) and Thomasson and colleagues (1991) examined the genotypes of the $ALDH_2$ locus of

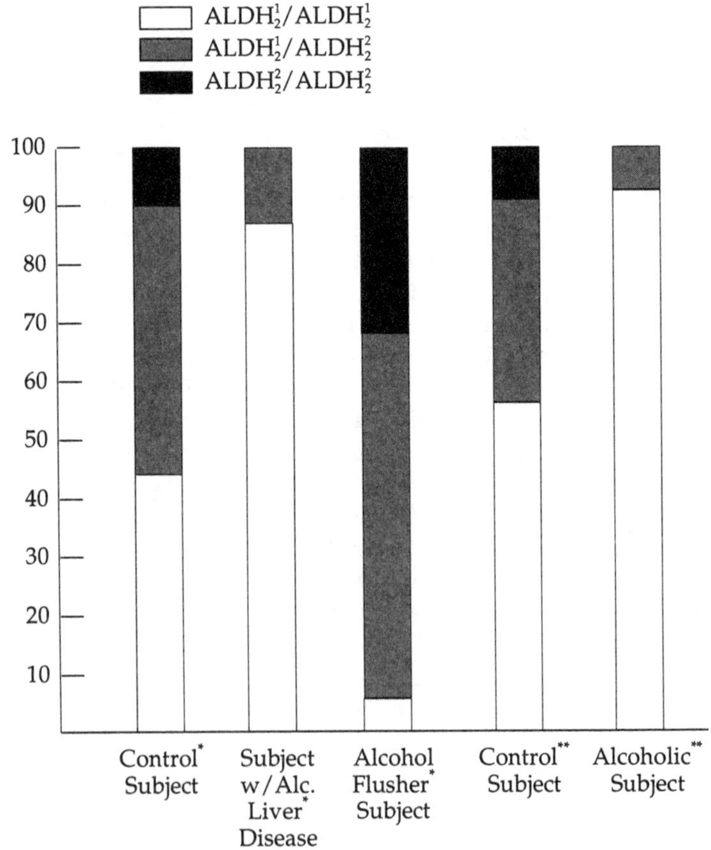

Figure 10–2. Genotypes of cytosolic aldehyde dehydrogenase gene ($ALDH_2$) in Japanese subjects with alcohol-related problems and in control subjects. * Data from Shibuya and Yoshida 1988a, 1988b and Shibuya et al. 1989. ** Data from Harada 1990.

Japanese and Chinese alcoholic patients and confirmed this conclusion.

The differences of ADH_2 genotypes between subjects who exhibit alcohol flushing and those who do not, and between patients with alcoholic liver diseases and control subjects, were not so remarkable as that of the $ALDH_2$ types (Table 10–5). We found no difference in the frequencies of the usual ADH_2^1 and atypical ADH_2^2 genes between patients with alcoholic liver disease and control subjects (Shibuya and Yoshida 1988b). In our earlier study involving a small number of samples, a lower frequency of the usual ADH_2^1 gene was found in alcohol flusher subjects than in nonflusher subjects (Shibuya et al. 1989). However, the later study using a large number of alcohol flusher subjects indicated that the difference is not significant (Table 10–5).

Thomasson and colleagues (1991) observed a somewhat higher frequency of the usual ADH_2^1 gene and the variant ADH_3^2 gene than the variant ADH_2^2 gene and the normal ADH_3^1 gene in Chinese alcoholic patients than in control subjects. They suggested that the more active enzymes produced by the ADH_2^2 and ADH_3^1 genes could elevate acetaldehyde level in the body and restrain alcohol-seeking tendencies.

Approximately 5%–8% of Caucasians exhibit alcohol flushing. In addition, about 6%–10% exhibit chlorpropamide-induced alcohol flushing (Baramuk et al. 1987; Ewing et al. 1974; Wilson et al. 1978; Wolff 1972). The characteristic seems to be a dominantly inherited trait. All Caucasians thus far examined are homozygous 1-1 in the $ALDH_2$ locus. Thus, the genetic background of Caucasians who exhibited alcohol flushing is different from that

Table 10–5. Genotypes of ADH_2 locus in Japanese subjects

	Genotypes			**Gene frequency**	
	1-1	**1-2**	**2-2**	ADH_2^1	ADH_2^2
Control subjects (*n* = 49)	4	20	25	0.29	0.71
Patients with alcoholic liver disease (*n* = 23)	3	6	14	0.26	0.74
Alcohol flusher subjects (*n* = 25)	2	9	14	0.26	0.74
Nonflusher subjects (*n* = 8)	0	4	4	0.25	0.75

of Asians. By examining the properties of the $ALDH_1$ isozyme existing in blood samples from Caucasian alcohol flusher subjects, two types of $ALDH_1$ variants were found (Yoshida et al. 1989). The enzyme deficiency and flushing character are coinherited in relatives of one of the probands. The physiological mechanism of alcohol flushing is not identical in Asians and Caucasians. Asian subjects who exhibit alcohol flushing have a pronounced rise in the blood acetaldehyde level and exhibit tachycardia, but these changes do not occur in $ALDH_1$-deficient Caucasian subjects who exhibit alcohol flushing (Ward et al. 1991).

The genotypes of American Indians have been a subject of interest. Both American Indians and Asians are of Mongoloid origin, and a high frequency of alcohol flushing has been observed in both populations (Wolff 1973). Unlike Asians, American Indians have a very high frequency of alcohol-related problems. It has been reported that American Indians and Canadian Indians show no (or a low) frequency of mitochondrial $ALDH_2$ deficiency, whereas approximately 40% of American Indians in South America lack $ALDH_2$ activity (Goedde et al. 1986; Zeiner et al. 1984). However, recent genotype analysis indicated that none of 28 American Indians from South America who were examined had the atypical Asian type $ALDH_2^2$ gene (O'Dowd et al. 1990). Should about 40% of American Indians in South America lack $ALDH_2$ activity, another defective mutant $ALDH_2$ gene, which differs from the atypical Asian type $ALDH_2^2$ gene, might exist at a high frequency in the American Indian population. Our research team determined the genotypes of both ADH_2 and $ALDH_2$ loci of American Indians and Canadian Indians and found that they do not have the Asian type ADH_2^2 and $ALDH_2^2$ genes in detectable frequency (< 2%) (A. Yoshida, unpublished data, April 1992).

CONCLUSION

It is now clear that Asians with the atypical Asian type $ALDH_2^2$ gene, in both homozygous and heterozygous status, are alcohol sensitive and are at very low risk for developing alcoholism and alcoholic liver diseases. The atypical $ALDH_2^2$ gene is a major "alcohol-rejecting" genetic factor in Asians. It is not necessary to reiterate that identification of "alcohol-seeking" gene(s) or "alcoholic" gene(s) is very important. Family pedigree studies and adoption studies have demonstrated significant hereditary contribution in type 2 alcoholism (Goodwin et al. 1973; Schuckit et al. 1972).

Linkage of alcoholism with the dopamine D_2 receptor locus on chromosome 11 was reported by two groups (Blum et al. 1990; Comings et al. 1991), but it was disputed by other groups (Bolos et al. 1990; Gelernter et al. 1991). A large-scale cooperative study for the search of "alcoholic" genes is currently being undertaken. The approach, which includes elaborate classifications of phenotypes of several hundred alcoholic subjects and linkage analysis of many candidate genes and enzymes with alcoholism of various phenotypes, is rational and orthodox.

I would like to point out some problems involved in the study of genetic abnormalities which should be considered. The simplest and the most straightforward genetic disorders are single-gene abnormalities that cause well-defined symptoms, such as the specific nucleotide base change in hemoglobin β gene that results in sickle cell anemia and the abnormality of phenylalanine hydroxylase that results in phenylketonuria. Even in these "simplest" of genetic disorders, the degree of severity of clinical symptoms differs widely among individual patients with the same defective gene. Some genetic diseases are far more complex. For example, the congenital nonspherocytic hemolytic anemia cannot be attributed to a single-gene abnormality. It is known that abnormalities of 16 different enzymes controlled by separate genes can cause the same clinical symptom (i.e., nonspherocytic hemolytic anemia). In comparison to the central nervous system that controls human behavior, red blood cells are very simple, and we probably already know most if not all of the enzymes involved in red cell metabolism and intermediate metabolites. Nevertheless, we cannot currently identify the genetic abnormalities in about 70% of patients.

In the case of alcoholism, even if a major alcoholic gene (or genes) should exist, expression of the symptom is expected to be strongly affected by other genetic, epigenetic, environmental, social, and psychological factors. Therefore, elaborate classifications of alcoholic phenotypes to select key core families, as proposed by the large-scale cooperative study, may not be beneficial, but in fact may cause additional confusion in the linkage analysis.

I propose a simpler expectant study of target subjects for the search of a major alcoholic gene or genes on the following basis. Asians with genotype $ALDH_2^1/ALDH_2^2$ or $ALDH_2^2$ $/ALDH_2^2$ are alcohol sensitive and have a tendency to reject drinking a large amount of alcohol because of their genetic background. Nevertheless, a small number of patients (5%–10%) with alcoholism or alcoholic liver diseases are heterozygous $ALDH_2^1/ALDH_2^2$ (Figure 10–2). These few exceptions must be associated with extremely strong "alcohol-seeking" tendencies, which overcome the effect of the "alcohol-rejecting" $ALDH_2^2$ gene. It is worthwhile to study the nature of this "alcohol-seeking" tendency, which may be related to a major "alcohol-seeking" gene or "alcoholic" gene.

REFERENCES

Baramuk JN, Murray RB, Mabbee WG: Naloxone, ethanol, and the chlorpropamide alcohol flush. Alcohol Clin Exp Res 11:518–520, 1987

Blum K, Noble EP, Sheridan PJ, et al: Allelic association of human dopamine D_2 receptor gene in alcoholism. JAMA 263:2055–2059, 1990

Bolos AM, Dean M, Lucas-Derse S, et al: Population and pedigree studies reveal a lack of association between the dopamine D_2 receptor gene and alcoholism. JAMA 264:3156–3160, 1990

Comings DE, Comings BG, Muhleman D, et al: The dopamine D_2 receptor locus as a modifying gene in neuropsychiatric disorders. JAMA 266:1793–1800, 1991

Duley JA, Harris O, Holmes RS: Analysis of human alcohol and aldehyde metabolizing isozymes by electrophoresis and isoelectric focusing. Alcohol Clin Exp Res 9:263–271, 1985

Eckey R, Agarwal DP, Saha N, et al: Detection and partial characterization of a variant cytosolic aldehyde dehydrogenase isozyme. Hum Genet 72:95–97, 1986

Ewing JA, Rouse BA, Pellizzari ED: Alcohol sensitivity and ethnic background. Am J Psychiatry 131:206–210, 1974

Frezza M, di Padora C, Pozzato G, et al: High blood alcohol levels in women: the role of decreased gastric alcohol dehydrogenase activity and first pass metabolism. N Engl J Med 322:95–99, 1990

Gelernter J, O'Malley S, Risch N, et al: No association between an allele at the D_2 dopamine receptor gene (DRD_2) and alcoholism. JAMA 266:1801–1807, 1991

Goedde HW, Agarwal DP, Harada S: Alcohol dehydrogenase polymorphism in North American, South American, and Mexican Indian populations. Am J Hum Genet 38:395–399, 1986

Goodwin DW, Schulsinger F, Hermansen L, Winokur G: Alcohol problems in adoptees raised apart from alcoholic biological parents. Arch Gen Psychiatry 28:238–243, 1973

Harada S: Genetic polymorphism of aldehyde dehydrogenase and its physiological significance to alcohol metabolism. Prog Clin Biol Res 344:289–291, 1990

Hopkinson DA, Santisteban I, Povey S, Smith M: Biochemical genetic analysis of human and rodent aldehyde dehydrogenase (ALDH). Alcohol 2:73–78, 1985

Hsu LC, Chang WC: Cloning and characterization of a new functional human aldehyde dehydrogenase gene. J Biol Chem 266:12257–12265, 1991

Hsu LC, Tani K, Fujiyoshi T, et al: Cloning of cDNAs for human aldehyde dehydrogenase 1 and 2. Proc Natl Acad Sci USA 82:3771–3775, 1985

Hsu LC, Bendel RE, Yoshida A: Direct detection of usual and atypical alleles on human aldehyde dehydrogenase-2 ($ALDH_2$) locus. Am J Hum Genet 41:996–1001, 1987

Hsu LC, Chang WC, Shibuya A, et al: Human stomach aldehyde dehydrogenase cDNA and genomic cloning, primary structure and expression in *E. coli*. J Biol Chem 267:3030–3037, 1992

Ikuta T, Shibuya A, Yoshida A: Direct determination of usual (Caucasian type) and atypical (Oriental type) alleles of class I human alcohol dehydrogenase-2 locus. Biochem Genet 26:519–525, 1988

Mizoi Y, Ijiri I, Tatsuno Y, et al: Relationship between facial flushing and blood acetaldehyde levels after alcohol intake. Pharmacol Biochem Behav 10:301–311, 1979

Moreno A, Parés X: Purification and characterization of a new alcohol dehydrogenase from human stomach. J Biol Chem 266:1128–1133, 1991

O'Dowd BF, Rothhammer F, Israel Y: Genotyping of mitochondrial aldehyde dehydrogenase locus of native South American Indians. Alcohol Clin Exp Res 14:531–533, 1990

Schuckit MA, Goodwin DW, Winokur G: A study of alcoholism in half-siblings. Am J Psychiatry 128:1132–1136, 1972

Shibuya A, Yoshida A: Frequency of the atypical aldehyde dehydrogenase-2 gene ($ALDH_2^2$) in Japanese and Caucasians. Am J Hum Genet 43:744–748, 1988a

Shibuya A, Yoshida A: Genotypes of alcohol metabolizing enzymes in Japanese with alcoholic liver disease: a strong association of the usual Caucasian type aldehyde dehydrogenase gene ($ALDH_2^1$) with the disease. Am J Hum Genet 43:744–748, 1988b

Shibuya A, Yasunami M, Yoshida A: Genotypes of alcohol dehydrogenase and aldehyde dehydrogenase loci in Japanese alcohol flushers and non-flushers. Hum Genet 82:14–16, 1989

Singh S, Fritz G, Fang B, et al: Inheritance of mitochondrial aldehyde dehydrogenase: genotyping in Chinese, Japanese and South Korean families reveals dominance of the mutant allele. Hum Genet 83:119–121, 1989

Thomasson HR, Edenberg HJ, Crabb DW, et al: Alcohol and aldehyde dehydrogenase genotypes and alcoholism in Chinese men. Am J Hum Genet 48:677–681, 1991

Ward R, Macpherson A, Warren-Perry M, et al: Biochemical and genetic studies in ALDH1-deficient subjects, in Alcoholism: A Molecular Perspective. Edited by Palmer TN. New York, Plenum, 1991, pp 139–143

Wilson JR, McClearn GE, Johnson RC: Ethnic variation in the use and effects of alcohol. Drug Alcohol Depend 3:147–151, 1978

Wolff PH: Ethnic difference in alcohol sensitivity. Science 175:449–450, 1972

Wolff PH: Vasomotor sensitivity to alcohol in diverse mongoloid population. Am J Hum Genet 25:193–199, 1973

Yasunami M, Chen CS, Yoshida A: A human alcohol dehydrogenase gene (ADH_6) encoding an additional class of isozyme. Proc Natl Acad Sci USA 88:7610–7614, 1991

Yin SJ, Cheng TC, Chang CP, et al: Human stomach alcohol and aldehyde dehydrogenase: a genetic model proposed for ALDH III isozymes. Biochem Genet 26:345–360, 1988

Yin SJ, Wang MF, Liao CS, Chen CM, Wu CW: Identification of a human stomach alcohol dehydrogenase with distinctive kinetic properties. Biochem Int 22:829–835, 1990

Yoshida A: A possible structural variant of human cytosolic aldehyde dehydrogenase with diminished enzyme activity. Am J Hum Genet 35:1115–1116, 1983

Yoshida A, Huang IY, Ikawa M: Molecular abnormality of an inactive aldehyde dehydrogenase variant commonly found in Orientals. Proc Natl Acad Sci USA 81:258–261, 1984

Yoshida A, Ward RJ, Peters TJ: Cytosolic aldehyde dehydrogenase ($ALDH_1$) variants found in alcohol flushers. Ann Hum Genet 53:1–7, 1989

Yoshida A, Shibuya A, Dave V, et al: Developmental changes of aldehyde dehydrogenase isozymes in human livers: mitochondrial $ALDH_2$ isozyme is expressed in fetal livers. Experientia 46:747–750, 1990

Yoshida A, Hsu LC, Yasunami M: Genetics of human alcohol-metabolizing enzymes. Prog Nucleic Acid Res Mol Biol 40:255–287, 1991

Zeiner HR, Girardot JM, Nichols N, et al: ALDH I isozyme deficiency among North American Indians (abstract). Proceedings of the 2nd Congress of the International Society for Biomedical Research on Alcoholism, 1984, p 129

Section III

Ethnicity and Psychobiology

Chapter 11

Ethnicity and Biological Markers

Russell E. Poland, Ph.D., and Keh-Ming Lin, M.D., M.P.H.

The influence of ethnicity on the etiology and expression of normal and abnormal biological processes has gained considerable attention during the past few years. Although great strides have been made in many areas of medicine in relation to ethnicity in general (Cruickshank and Beevers 1989; Polednak 1989), considerably fewer advances have been made in the clinical neurosciences. For example, there is no section on ethnicity and psychopharmacology or psychobiology in *Psychopharmacology, The Third Generation of Progress* (Meltzer 1987), a 1,780-page treatise about the domain of psychopharmacology. Although awareness of ethnicity and psychobiological issues is growing in the scientific community (Lawson 1986), it still has not received the attention it merits.

Unlike other branches of medicine, progress in psychiatry in general has long been impeded by the absence of "objective" laboratory tests (Cowen and Wood 1991; Freedman 1987; Schuckit 1988) or "biological markers." Although so-called biological markers have been described for a variety of psychiatric disorders including, but not limited to, depression, schizophrenia, panic disorder, and posttraumatic stress disorders, there is a dearth of information as to whether these measures are ethnically valid.

Supported in part by National Institute of Mental Health (NIMH) MH34471 (Dr. Poland), the Research Center on the Psychobiology of Ethnicity MH47193 (Drs. Lin and Poland), NIMH Research Scientist Development Award MH00534 (Dr. Poland), and by National Institute of Health Clinical Research Center Grant RR 00425.

In this chapter, we review the limited data on the influence of ethnicity on psychobiological measures. Data from subjects with psychiatric disorders and from control subjects of different ethnic backgrounds are also presented.

ETHNICITY AND BIOLOGICAL MARKERS OF PSYCHIATRIC DISORDERS

Depression

One of the most studied biological markers of depression is the dexamethasone suppression test (DST; Carroll et al. 1981). The DST response has been reported to be abnormal in approximately 50% of patients with major depression, although this value can vary considerably. Escobar and colleagues (1984) reported that "Anglo" subjects had more than twice the rate of DST nonsuppression compared with African-American and Hispanic patients, all of whom were diagnosed as having a major depressive disorder using DSM-III criteria (American Psychiatric Association 1980). The percentage nonsuppression for 33 "Anglo," 12 African-American, and 8 Hispanic patients was 58%, 25%, and 0%, respectively (χ^2 = 9.91, df = 2, P =.007). Unfortunately, no control subjects were studied; therefore, specificity and diagnostic confidence for each ethnic group could not be calculated. In a study of 40 definite endogenous depressive patients and 40 age-, sex-, and race-matched control subjects, 15 patients (37.5%) were classified as DST nonsuppressors (Rubin et al. 1987). Five of the 40 patients were African-American, and all 5 were suppressors, as were their 5 matched control subjects. In a small study by Lawson (1986) on five Hispanic major depressive patients diagnosed according to DSM-III criteria, none showed an abnormal DST response. In contrast, De La Fuente and Amor (1986) reported a DST nonsuppression rate of 36% and a specificity of 91% in their study of Hispanic patients. However, no other ethnic groups were studied at their site, nor was it clear as to how the researchers determined sensitivity and specificity.

A World Health Organization (WHO) collaborative study on depression has included a DST as part of its study protocol (Coppen et al. 1984). Thirteen sites participated in the study, and a total of 541 subjects with major depression and 220 control subjects were administered the 1.0-mg DST (Carroll et al. 1981). All samples were analyzed for cortisol in the same laboratory. DST nonsuppression ranged from 15% (8 of 54) in Moscow to 71% (10 of 14) in Copenhagen. The Asian sites, Nagasaki and Sapporo, had the next two lowest rates of DST nonsuppression, 21% (6 of 28) and 23% (12 of 52), respectively, followed by the North African site, which had a 25% (3 of 12) nonsuppression rate. The American site (California) reported a 42% (11 of 26) rate of nonsuppression. Although the two Japanese sites showed low rates of nonsuppression, inpatient DST studies conducted in Taiwan have shown "satisfactory" nonsuppression rates ranging from 59% to 67% (Hwu et al. 1981, 1985). However, the outpatients examined in one of these studies (Hwu et al. 1985) revealed an extremely low nonsuppression rate of 7%, even though the symptom profiles of these outpatients appeared to be similar to those of the inpatients.

Another biological abnormality observed in patients with major depression—one that occurs even more frequently than DST nonsuppression—is shortened rapid eye movement (REM) sleep latency (cf. Poland et al. 1989; Rush et al. 1982). A collaborative cross-cultural study by the WHO (Mendelwicz and Kerkhofs 1991) reported on sleep electroencephalogram (EEG) abnormalities in subjects with major depression studied at eight different sites in Europe, North America, and Asia. As a group, the depressed patients showed sleep-continuity disturbances, shortened REM latency, and increased REM density compared to control subjects. However, it was not clear if there were quantitative or qualitative differences in these measures at the individual sites, as had been found for DST responses described previously.

Schizophrenia and Other Psychobiological Disorders

To our knowledge there are only a few reports describing ethnic differences of biological measures in schizophrenic patients. As reviewed by Lawson (1986), there have indeed been sporadic reports that suggested significant ethnic differences in some of the biological markers currently under investigation. For example, platelet serotonin (5-HT) concentrations were found to be increased in African-American schizophrenic patients compared to African-American control subjects, with no differences found between Caucasian patients and Caucasian control subjects (Jackman et al. 1983). African-American and Caucasian patients with affective disorder also showed no differences. Ethnic contrasts in platelet and lymphocyte monoamine oxidase (MAO) activity also have been reported (Bridge et al. 1983; DeLisi et al. 1980). A significant correlation was found between low MAO activity and persistence of schizophrenic symptomatology among Caucasians but not among African-Americans. In addition, an increased HLA-A2 antigen frequency has been seen among African-American schizophrenic patients as compared to their Caucasian counterparts (Luchins et al. 1980). Because many of the above-mentioned biological measures have all been proposed as possible markers for schizophrenia, the ethnic differences suggested here are intriguing and worthy of more careful attention.

To our knowledge, cross-ethnic studies of biological markers in subjects with other psychiatric disorders have not been reported. The single study of alcoholism showed that carbohydrate-deficient transferrin was higher in African-American alcoholic patients than in Caucasian alcoholic patients who consumed comparable amounts of ethanol (Behrens et al. 1988).

Control Subjects

Not only are there ethnic differences in various measures related to psychiatric disorders, but there also are reports of ethnic differences for a variety of biological measures in control subjects (cf. Lawson 1986). For example, black control subjects have been reported to have higher basal lymphocyte cyclic adenosine monophosphate (cAMP) levels, as well as a greater response to isoprenaline, suggesting an increased number or sensitivity of $beta_2$-adrenoceptors (Venter et al. 1985). Also related to the immune system is the observation that lymphocytes obtained from African-American control subjects show significantly lower interleukin (IL)-2 production to phytohemagglutinin stimulation than do Caucasian control subjects (Ganguli and Rabin 1989). Serum creatinine phosphokinase (CPK) activity also has been found to be significantly higher among healthy blacks compared to Caucasians (Meltzer 1971), and it also has been shown that erythrocyte catechol-O-methyltransferase activity is significantly greater in Asians than in Caucasians (Rivera-Calimlim and Reilly 1983).

There are also data suggesting that ethnicity can influence various physiological and pharmacologic responses in vivo. Venter and colleagues (1984) reported that the heart rate response to atropine was significantly greater in African-American control subjects than in Caucasians. However, the heart rate response to propranolol was comparable, both at rest and following administration of atropine. These results suggest that the contribution of parasympathetic tone to resting heart rate is greater in African-Americans than in Caucasians. In contrast to the increased sensitivity of African-Americans to atropine, the reduction in heart rate following metoprolol was less in African-Americans than in Caucasians, suggesting that African-American subjects have an increase in $beta_1$-receptor–coupled activity (Rutledge et al. 1989). The mydriatic response to systemically administered atropine has been shown to be less in African-Americans than in Caucasians (Garde et al. 1978).

The differential sensitivity of cholinergic systems among ethnic groups can be inferred further from the findings of Lu and colleagues (1990) in relation to the cardiovascular response to the Valsalva maneuver. Although resting blood pressure was found to be significantly higher in African-Americans than in Caucasians or Asians, the fall in systolic blood pressure from baseline during the Valsalva maneuver was significantly greater in Asians and African-Americans than in Caucasians. The reduction in carotid artery blood flow velocity during the Valsalva maneuver was significantly less in African-Americans.

DISCUSSION

General Issues

With the phenomenal and increasingly accelerating growth of various branches of the neurosciences, including sleep research, neuroimaging, receptor assays, neuroendocrinology, and the measurement of neurotransmitters and their metabolites, our understanding of the neurobiological substrates and correlates of various psychiatric disorders is rapidly expanding. Results from these research studies have identified putative biological markers for the various psychiatric conditions. Although the specificity and meaning of most of these findings are still being debated, it is reasonable to expect that some of these research efforts will eventually lead to the establishment of "tests" that are clinically useful. Unfortunately, so far ethnicity has received negligible or at most only peripheral attention by researchers engaged in these efforts.

It is clear that few studies have been performed on the influence of ethnicity on psychobiological processes, with many of the studies that have been done being only preliminary in nature. This is lamentable for both theoretical and practical reasons. At the practical level, the clinical applicability and the criteria adopted for these biological "tests" should not be transported en masse from one ethnic group to another; rather, they should be evaluated carefully for each group. At the theoretical level, cross-ethnic comparison and validation could and should be used to clarify the significance and meaning of biological changes associated with major psychiatric syndromes.

One of the promises of using biological measures for differential diagnosis is that they might prove to be a culture-free means of assessment. Investigations in this direction, while still preliminary in nature, could have profound implications in cross-cultural research in the future. If biological markers can indeed be used in this fashion, then they will vastly improve our ability to understand how sociocultural as well as other environmental (nonbiological) variables influence symptom manifestation, clinical course, treatment response, and long-term outcome in patients with a similar kind of disability, as determined by biological parameters. Thus, the relationship between ethnicity and psychobiology is an important variable that needs to be addressed systematically. It should be noted that a difference in a biological measure between ethnic groups should not be misconstrued to denote a "genetic" basis for the difference. Although this might be the case, as it can be for the metabolism of alcohol (see Chapter 10), it is conceivable that other factors such as demographics, socioeconomic class, and/or environment could contribute significantly to the observed differences.

Potential Mechanisms for Ethnic Differences

As mentioned in Chapter 2, childhood experience can play a key role in the development and maturation of the central nervous system (CNS), producing "hardwired" alterations in the structure-function relationships of the brain in the adult organism. For example, numerous preclinical studies have shown that animals exposed to various stressors (e.g., handling, restraint) during early development manifest abnormal hypothalamic-pituitary-adrenal (HPA) responses to a variety of provocations as adults (Hamamura and Onaka 1989; Meaney et al. 1989; Peters 1982). Thus, by analogy, the effect of ethnicity on the DST response could be due to cross-cultural factors that occurred during development and not necessarily to genetic differences or differences among ethnic groups in the neurobiological underpinning of the disorder. It is interesting to speculate that these same factors could also be important determinants as to why only some patients with major depression, ethnicity notwithstanding, show upregulation of the HPA axis during a major depressive episode.

Although the results of the few available studies support our hypothesis of ethnic influences on biological marker presentation, methodological issues might also have contributed to the results. For example, none of the studies mentioned here measured serum dexamethasone concentrations, which we (Poland et al. 1987) and others have shown can markedly influence the DST response. It is well known that different ethnic groups metabolize drugs at markedly different rates; therefore, the reduced metabolism or bioavailability of dexamethasone (due to genetic and/or environmental factors) could have contributed to the differences in the nonsuppression rates. Noncompliance (not taking dexamethasone as instructed) also might have contributed to the inconsistent results—although this would increase DST nonsuppression rates that, if anything, have tended to be lower in Asians, blacks, and Hispanics as compared to Caucasians. Compliance is a variable that also can be addressed by measuring serum dexamethasone concentrations. To our knowledge, other than the DST, no direct assessment of the status of HPA axis has been reported in depressed patients in relation to ethnicity. Because so many factors can affect the DST response, more direct assessments of the HPA axis appear warranted. It should be noted that variations in the patient evaluation procedures, absence of appropriate control groups, and differences in time of blood collection, processing, and analytic methodology also could have contributed to the inconsistent DST findings.

In a number of studies (cf. Lin et al. 1991; Mendoza et al. 1991; Strickland et al. 1991), data suggest that there might be ethnic differences in the status of cholinergic systems in both control subjects and in subjects with certain psychiatric disorders. If so, this factor also could contribute to the observed differences in the DST response and possibly in REM sleep measures as well, both of which are influenced strongly by cholinergic systems (Dilsaver and Coffman 1989; cf. Janowsky et al. 1972; Poland et al. 1989).

An interesting observation in Asians is that catechol-O-methyltransferase activity, associated with one of the important enzymes involved in the metabolism of amines, has been found to be significantly increased in Asians (Pilipinos, Chinese, and Thais) as compared to Caucasians (Rivera-Calimlim and Reilly 1983). Because dysfunction of amine systems has been implicated in the pathogenesis of both schizophrenia and affective disorders, this finding is not without potentially profound ramifications. Whether such differences occur in blacks or Hispanics is not known, although data obtained from peripheral measures suggest that they might (Bridge et al. 1983; DeLisi et al. 1980; Jackman et al. 1983).

Implications of Similarities Versus Differences

In addition to the reported differences in biological measures between schizophrenic patients of divergent ethnicity, there also are data showing similarities. It has been reported that Asian schizophrenic patients with higher plasma homovanillic acid (HVA) concentrations show a better response to haloperidol treatment than do Asian patients with lower plasma HVA concentrations (Chang et al. 1990). These findings are comparable to those found with Caucasian schizophrenic patients, suggesting that the neurochemical underpinnings of schizophrenia for these two ethnic groups are similar, at least in regard to this measure. However, a significant correlation between plasma HVA and symptom severity was not found in the Taiwan study, although it has been reported at the Western sites (Davidson and Davis 1988; Davis et al. 1985; Pickar et al. 1984). This difference might be related to ethnic differences in symptom presentation—differences that could be used as a tool to tease apart those symptoms that are "core" symptoms versus those that might only be related peripherally to the disorder.

These results also help to illustrate another critical issue. As we discussed, the frequency of DST nonsuppression in depressed patients was found to be only 21% and 23% in Nagasaki and Sapporo, Japan, respectively. However, the rates of nonsuppression in Taiwan were comparable to that found in Western countries: more than 50% (Hwu et al. 1981, 1985). Thus, the similarity of the plasma HVA data between Caucasians and Asians in Taiwan should not be overinterpreted. All Asians are not alike; nor are all blacks, Caucasians, or Hispanics.

SUMMARY

Our understanding of neurobiology of psychiatric disorders is just beginning. Most of the studies performed to date have utilized Caucasian subjects, although Caucasians are a minority population in the world. Ethnicity is an important issue in such studies for a number of reasons:

1. The presence or absence of biological markers in different ethnic groups with comparable psychiatric disorders should provide important data regarding the universality of the pathophysiologic underpinnings of the disorders.
2. Cross-cultural confirmation of the associations between these biological markers and psychiatric syndromes should help to establish the validity (and clinical utility) of these "tests."
3. The inclusion of some of these biological markers in cross-ethnic studies might help to ensure the comparability of patients recruited for these studies.

The results of such studies will have important clinical applications as well as implications for basic research and will help to guide future research in the area of biological markers and psychiatric disorders.

REFERENCES

American Psychiatric Association: Diagnostic and Statistical Manual of Mental Disorders, 3rd Edition. Washington, DC, American Psychiatric Association, 1980

Behrens UJ, Worner TM, Braly LF, et al: Carbohydrate-deficient transferrin, a marker for chronic alcohol consumption in different ethnic population. Alcohol Clin Exp Res 12:427–432, 1988

Bridge P, Jeste DV, Wise CD, et al: Schizophrenic outcome in late life: symptom state and platelet monoamine oxidase activity. Psychiatr Res 11:91–97, 1983

Carroll BJ, Feinberg M, Greden J, et al: A specific laboratory test for the diagnosis of melancholia: standardization, validation, and clinical utility. Arch Gen Psychiatry 38:15–22, 1981

Chang WH, Chen TY, Lin SK, et al: Plasma catecholamine metabolites in schizophrenics: evidence for the two-subtype concept. Biol Psychiatry 27:510–518, 1990

Coppen A, Metcalfe M, Harwood J, et al: WHO collaborative study on the use of the dexamethasone suppression test as a biological indicator of depressive illness. Clin Neuropharmacol 7:226–227, 1984

Cowen PJ, Wood AJ: Biological markers of depression. Psychol Med 21:831–836, 1991

Cruickshank JK, Beevers DG: Ethnic Factors in Health and Disease. London, Wright, 1989

Davidson M, Davis K: A comparison of plasma homovanillic acid concentrations in schizophrenic patients and normal controls. Arch Gen Psychiatry 45:561–563, 1988

Davis KL, Davidson M, Mohs RC, et al: Plasma homovanillic acid concentrations and the severity of schizophrenic illness. Science 227:1601–1602, 1985

De La Fuente JR, Amor JS: Does ethnicity affect DST results? (letter). Am J Psychiatry 143:275–276, 1986

DeLisi L, Neckers LM, Staub RA, et al: Lymphocyte monoamine oxidase activity and chronic schizophrenia. Psychiatry Res 2:179–186, 1980

Dilsaver SC, Coffman JA: Cholinergic hypothesis of depression: a reappraisal. J Clin Psychopharmacol 9:173–179, 1989

Escobar JI, Mendoza R, Stimmel G, et al: The DST in a large outpatient clinic: its diagnostic and predictive significance. Psychopharmacol Bull 20:89–92, 1984

Freedman DX: Strategies for research in biological psychiatry, in Psychopharmacology: The Third Generation of Progress. Edited by Meltzer HY. New York, Raven, 1987, pp 23–31

Ganguli R, Rabin BS: Differences in interleukin-2 production in Blacks and Whites. N Engl J Med 320:349, 1989

Garde JF, Aston R, Endler GC, et al: Racial mydriatic response to belladonna premedication. Anesth Analg 57:572–576, 1978

Hamamura M, Onaka T: Pre-weaning handling reduces adrenocorticotropin response to novel but not to noxious stimuli in adult rats. Neurosci Lett 105:312–315, 1989

Hwu HG, Rudorfer MV, Clayton PJ: Dexamethasone suppression test and subtypes of depression (letter). Arch Gen Psychiatry 38:363, 1981

Hwu HG, Chen TY, Yang YY: The clinical diagnostic value of dexamethasone suppression test in depressive illness. Ann Acad Med Singapore 14:104–109, 1985

Jackman H, Luchins D, Meltzer HY: Platelet serotonin levels in schizophrenia: relationship to race and psychopathology. Biol Psychiatry 18:887–902, 1983

Janowsky DS, El-Yousef MK, Davis JM, et al: A cholinergic-adrenergic hypothesis for mania and depression. Lancet 2:632–635, 1972

Lawson WB: Racial and ethnic factors in psychiatric research. Hosp Community Psychiatry 37:50–54, 1986

Lin KM, Poland RE, Smith MW, et al: Pharmacokinetic and other related factors affecting psychotropic responses in Asians. Psychopharmacol Bull 27:427–439, 1991

Lu ZY, Metzger BL, Therrien B: Ethnic differences in physiological responses associated with the Valsalva maneuver. Res Nurs Health 13:9–15, 1990

Luchins D, Torrey EF, Weinberger DR, et al: HLA antigens in schizophrenia: differences between patients with and without evidence of brain atrophy. Br J Psychiatry 136:243–248, 1980

Meaney MJ, Aitken DH, Viau V, et al: Neonatal handling alters adrenocortical negative feedback sensitivity and hippocampal type II glucocorticoid receptor binding in the rat. Neuroendocrinology 50:597–604, 1989

Meltzer HY: Factors affecting serum creatine phosphokinase levels in the general population: the role of race, activity and age. Clin Chim Acta 33:165–172, 1971

Meltzer HY (ed): Psychopharmacology: The Third Generation of Progress. New York, Raven, 1987
Mendelwicz J, Kerkhofs M: Sleep electroencephalography in depressive illness: a collaborative study by the World Health Organization. Br J Psychiatry 159:505–509, 1991
Mendoza R, Smith MV, Poland RE, et al: Ethnic psychopharmacology: the Hispanic and Native American perspective. Psychopharmacol Bull 27:449–461, 1991
Peters DAV: Prenatal stress: effects on brain biogenic amine and plasma corticosterone levels. Pharmacol Biochem Behav 17:721–725, 1982
Pickar D, Labarca R, Linnoila M, et al: Neuroleptic-induced decrease in plasma homovanillic acid and antipsychotic activity in schizophrenic patients. Science 225:954–957, 1984
Poland RE, Rubin RT, Lesser IM, et al: Neuroendocrine aspects of primary endogenous depression, II: serum dexamethasone concentrations and hypothalamic-pituitary-adrenal cortical activity as determinants of the dexamethasone suppression test response. Arch Gen Psychiatry 44:790–795, 1987
Poland RE, Tondo L, Trelease R, et al: Differential effects of scopolamine on nocturnal cortisol secretion, sleep architecture and REM latency in normal volunteers: relation to sleep and cortisol abnormalities in depression. Biol Psychiatry 25:403–412, 1989
Polednak AP: Racial and Ethnic Differences in Disease. New York, Oxford University Press, 1989
Rivera-Calimlim L, Reilly DK: Difference in erythrocyte catechol-O-methyltransferase activity between Orientals and Caucasians: difference in levodopa tolerance. Clin Pharmacol Ther 35:804–809, 1983
Rubin RT, Poland RE, Lesser IM, et al: Neuroendocrine aspects of primary endogenous depression, I: cortisol secretory dynamics in patients and matched controls. Arch Gen Psychiatry 44:328–336, 1987
Rush AJ, Giles DE, Roffwarg HP, et al: Sleep EEG and DST findings in outpatients with unipolar major depression. Biol Psychiatry 17:327–340, 1982
Rutledge DR, Steinberg J, Cardozo L: Racial differences in drug response: isoproterenol effects on heart rate following intravenous metoprolol. Clin Pharmacol Ther 45:380–386, 1989
Schuckit MA: Trait and state markers of a predisposition to psychopathology, in Psychiatry, Vol 3. Edited by Michels R. Philadelphia, PA, JB Lippincott, 1988, pp 1–19
Strickland RL, Ranganath V, Lin KM, et al: Psychopharmacologic considerations in the treatment of Black American populations. Psychopharmacol Bull 27:441–448, 1991

Venter CP, Joubert PH, Strydom WJ: Ethnic differences in response to pharmacological denervation of the heart. IRCS Medical Science 12:963–964, 1984

Venter CP, Daya S, Joubert PH, et al: Ethnic differences in human lymphocytic cyclic AMP production after isoprenaline stimulation and propranolol blockade. Br J Clin Pharmacol 19:187–190, 1985

Chapter 12

Biopsychosocial Perspective on Depression in African-Americans

Hector F. Myers, Ph.D.

American psychiatry has been struggling for decades to resolve questions about the relative significance of ethnicity and culture as sources of variability in the experience and expression of psychiatric disorders, especially mood disorders. Continued interest in this issue is justified by the growing diversity of the population of the United States, now estimated to be about 20% non-Caucasian. According to the most recent census (Bureau of the Census 1990), the population of the United States in 1980 included 12.1% African-Americans, 9.0% Hispanics, 2.9% Asians, and 0.8% American Indians.

Although current epidemiologic evidence indicates that there are few significant ethnic group differences in the prevalence of mood disorders, especially depression (Robins 1991; Robins et al. 1984), ethnic minority scholars have long argued that our conceptual models, diagnostic tools, and treatment approaches are inadequate to the task of identifying, diagnosing, and effectively treating psychiatric disorders in African-Americans and other ethnic groups (Lawson 1986; Neighbors et al. 1989; Sue 1988; Williams 1986). In addition, the demands on public mental health facilities to treat the growing numbers of economically marginalized, multiethnic patients underscore the need for focused scholarly attention to these questions (Cheung 1991; Cheung and Snowden 1990; President's Commission on Mental

---

Supported in part by NIGMS/MBRS Grant GM8140-16 and by NIMH Grant MH47193 to the Research Center on the Psychobiology of Ethnicity. The author thanks Masai Minters and Nabil Jouni, M.D., for their assistance in obtaining the literature on which this chapter is based.

Health 1978; Richards and Gottfredson 1985; Taube and Barrett 1985).

In this chapter, I tackle only one aspect of this problem. I review and discuss the available epidemiologic and clinical evidence on African-American–Caucasian differences in the experience and expression of depressive disorders. I then offer a biopsychosocial perspective to account for these differences and suggest that a multidimensional perspective be used to guide future research on this question.

THE PROBLEM OF ETHNICITY AND CULTURE IN PSYCHOPATHOLOGY

The first major obstacle we face in understanding ethnicity and culture as potential contributors to differences in health and vulnerability to illness is in how we conceptualize these factors. Too often, as noted by Cooper (1984, 1991) and others (Crews and Bindon 1991; Gould 1981; Montagu 1945), we treat ethnic groups as biologically distinct groups and ignore the genetic and biological heterogeneity within groups (see also Chapter 1). This reinforces the error of assuming that observed differences between groups are due to biological differences between those groups. We cannot ignore the possibility that some group differences may be due to such biological differences; however, we concur with Crews and Bindon (1991) that "race is a sociological construct that is poorly correlated with any measurable biological or cultural phenomenon . . . [while] ethnicity is a sociocultural construct that is often, if not always, coextensive with discernible features of a group" (p. 42). Therefore, we believe that the available evidence makes a stronger case for interpreting reported differences in symptom expression and in response to psychoactive agents (see Strickland et al. 1991 for a review of the evidence on African-Americans) as biological consequences of cultural, social status, and life-style differences between ethnic groups rather than as the products of genetically determined group differences. This is the perspective that informs the analysis presented in this chapter.

The debate over the role of ethnicity and culture in psychopathology centers around two sets of questions about how these factors might contribute to differences in the occurrence and in the presentation of clinical symptoms of disorders such as depression, and how these differences, in turn, might complicate diagnostic decisions and contribute to diagnostic errors. The first set of questions is conceptual in nature. Investigators have frequently asked: Do ethnicity and culture confer differential vulnerability to or protection from mood disorders? Furthermore, are such differences attributable to identifiable biological, cultural, or socioecologic factors that influence how groups experience and/or express psychiatric distress?

The second set of questions, on the other hand, is more pragmatic and methodological in nature. Here we struggle with other questions: How valid and reliable are our standard diagnostic systems, measures, and procedures? Are clinical judgments significantly more unreliable and inaccurate when we diagnose mood disorders in patients from different cultural or ethnic backgrounds, either because of ethnic biases, cross-cultural unfamiliarity, or both (Baskin et al. 1981; Edwards 1982; Fellini 1989)?

Dozens of articles have been written to address these issues, especially in relation to African-American–Caucasian differences in the prevalence of depressive disorders, and the hypothesized greater vulnerability of African-Americans to misdiagnosis resulting from the ethnic, gender, and socioeconomic status (SES) biases of clinicians (Adebimpe 1981; Adebimpe et al. 1979; Hanson and Klerman 1974; Neighbors et al. 1989). Investigators have attempted to answer the core questions noted previously by debating the evidence for and against three competing hypotheses about what accounts for African-American–Caucasian differences in depression observed:

1. That symptom presentation is essentially the same across ethnic groups; therefore, differences in the prevalence of disorders are real and reflect differences in biological and/or psychosocial vulnerability;
2. That symptom presentation is the same across groups, and any observed group differences in prevalence rates are artifacts created by limitations in the diagnostic systems and/or by diagnostician bias; or alternatively

3. That there are some differences between groups in pattern of symptom expression, and that some of the observed differences in prevalence rates are real, whereas others may be distorted by instrumentation and/or diagnostician biases.

Unfortunately, despite decades of debate on these issues, there continues to be little evidence on which to base firm conclusions in support of any of these competing hypotheses. Consistent with hypothesis 3, we suspect that there are both similarities and differences in symptom expression across ethnic groups and that diagnostic biases do operate to inflate or deflate the rates of reported disorders in various groups. We also suspect that these artifacts vary in their salience across studies, across ethnic groups, and across types of psychiatric disorders. Given this state of affairs, therefore, we believe that current studies of ethnic issues in psychiatry might be more productive if they focused on specific hypothesized sources of ethnic group differences (e.g., differences in biological or psychosocial vulnerability in specific disorders, variability in symptom expression in specific disorders, etc.).

AFRICAN-AMERICAN–CAUCASIAN DIFFERENCES IN DEPRESSION

Our research group has been especially intrigued by some of the reported ethnic differences in mood disorders, and the etiologic and therapeutic implications of such differences (Lin et al. 1986). Specifically, we have been interested in the evidence reported in previous studies that suggest differences between African-Americans and Caucasians in risk for depression, in the prevalence of depression, in the pattern of symptom expression, and in response to pharmacologic intervention. For example, several studies have reported that African-American unipolar depressed patients report more worry, muscular tension, general anxiety, and autonomic symptoms than Caucasians (Fabrega et al. 1988; Simon et al. 1973; Uhlenhuth and Paykel 1973) and that clinically depressed African-American patients are typically more negative, express more anger and hostility, and make more suicidal threats and gestures than depressed Caucasians (Derogatis et al.

1971; Raskin et al. 1975; Tonks et al. 1970). African-American unipolar and bipolar patients have also been described as reporting greater use of alcohol and drugs (e.g., cocaine) and having a greater family history of alcohol abuse than their Caucasian counterparts (Galanter et al. 1988; Heizer 1975; Warheit et al. 1973). This evidence suggests that both differences in symptom expression and in the involvement of cofactors that complicate the clinical picture may be operative. However, how these issues can be effectively distinguished to improve diagnostic accuracy and the effectiveness of treatment remains a challenge for both researchers and clinicians.

The issue of possible differences between African-Americans and Caucasians in vulnerability to a variety of biological and psychosocial factors that confer risk for depression has also been raised. For example, several studies have identified African-Americans as being exposed to disproportionately higher socioeconomic stresses and as likely to experience higher levels of psychological distress due to the combined effects of ethnicity and lower social class (Kessler and Neighbors 1986). This higher exposure to stressful environments is believed to confer higher risk for disorders such as depression that involve feelings of hopelessness, anger, frustration, perceived lack of control, and restricted resources for coping (Abramson et al. 1978; Dressler 1986; Dressler and Badger 1985; Kessler et al. 1985). These findings suggest that different sociocultural processes may be operating among various racial and ethnic groups to account for differential vulnerability to depression.

However, questions have been raised about the quality of the evidence in support of these hypotheses. For example, recent epidemiologic studies (Somervell et al. 1989; Weissman et al. 1988) failed to identify consistent ethnic differences in vulnerability to depression when gender and other cofactors are considered (e.g., substance use, low SES). On the other hand, studies of symptom presentation have yielded mixed results (Adebimpe et al. 1982; Zung et al. 1988). Thus, when taken as a whole, there seems to be suggestive evidence of some African-American–Caucasian differences in symptom expression in mood disorders, but little consistent evidence of either greater prevalence or greater vulnerability to depression.

AFRICAN-AMERICAN–CAUCASIAN DIFFERENCES IN COMORBID RISK FOR DEPRESSION

Although the evidence for consistent ethnic group differences in depression remains mixed, there is strong evidence that these groups differ in the prevalence of comorbid factors, especially across gender and social classes. These differences add to the problems of accurately diagnosing and treating depressive disorders across ethnic groups (Galanter et al. 1988). For example, the evidence seems to indicate greater prevalence of substance use in African-American men and women compared to Caucasians. This difference is especially evident between African-American and Caucasian women. However, social class is an important mediator, with these differences evident mainly among lower SES groups (Lawson 1986; Warheit et al. 1987; Williams 1986).

In addition, there is a growing body of evidence of ethnic differences in response to psychotropic medication (Lin et al. 1986; Raskin and Crook 1975; Wood and Zhou 1991; Ziegler and Biggs 1977), which suggests that there may be important ethnic group differences in the way biopsychosocial contributors in psychiatric disorders are interacting. For example, a review of ethnic differences in pharmacokinetics of tricyclic antidepressants (TCAs) and lithium by Strickland and colleagues (1991) indicates that African-Americans respond to TCAs and lithium differently than Caucasians do. Their review of the available evidence on TCAs indicates that African-Americans tend to have higher plasma TCA levels and to respond better and faster to TCAs, but they experience more toxic side effects of these drugs than Caucasians. Similarly, research on lithium indicates that African-American patients evidence less efficient cell membrane sodium-lithium countertransport and higher red blood cell (RBC)/plasma lithium ratios, and they may excrete lithium slower than Caucasians do. The latter complements the evidence of greater sodium retention and greater salt sensitivity in African-Americans, which is believed to be a genetically determined diathesis for hypertension (Blaustein and Grim 1991). If these findings are confirmed in more carefully designed and methodologically rigorous prospective studies, then the justification for considering ethnicity in prescribing these mood-altering agents will have been firmly established.

Therefore, although the evidence of differences in depression between African-Americans and Caucasians is provocative, this does not seem to be the most interesting research direction to pursue at this time. A more productive course of action would be to take a more within-group focus and to investigate the most promising etiologic and treatment hypotheses in the field in carefully selected samples of African-American subjects. Such an approach would help us to identify subgroups of African-Americans that differ in biological and psychosocial vulnerability to depression. We would then be able to test whether depression in these subgroups might be influenced by different etiologic factors and to then follow a different course and require different therapeutic strategies.

Also, because both biological and psychosocial factors have been implicated in mood disorders, we believe that this research would be greatly enhanced by using more integrative approaches that could test the interactive effects of both sources of influence. For example, a recent survey of the literature by our group failed to identify any studies that tested any of the major biological hypotheses about the etiology of depression in African-Americans, despite all of the empirical evidence implicating biochemical dysregulation in mood disorders. Also, despite the popular view that low-income African-Americans and other minorities are at enhanced risk for depression and similar disorders because of chronic socioecologic stresses, few if any studies have investigated any of the major psychosocial hypotheses regarding the onset and severity of depression in these populations. Finally, with the widespread abuse of addicting substances in inner-city communities, especially among African-American men, clinicians treating these patients often confront the problem of comorbidity of substance use in their depressed patients. Nevertheless, few if any studies have investigated whether the pattern of symptoms, disease course, response to treatment, or long-term outcomes of depression in African-Americans differ in cases of concurrent substance use.

Although the debate over the question of whether African-

Americans and Caucasians differ in vulnerability to depression and in response to antidepressants continues unabated, important limitations in our conceptualization and treatment of depressive disorders in African-Americans still evade our attention. Foremost among these is the almost exclusive reliance of clinicians on ethnic comparison studies as the basis for investigating depression in African-Americans. Although ethnic comparisons provide some useful insights, they also limit the types of questions that can be investigated and reinforce the error of treating African-Americans and Caucasians as if they were homogeneous groups. In addition, the findings from such studies are often limited by methodological deficits due to sample size, sample representativeness, or assessment and diagnostic tools used.

A less apparent but equally significant deficit is our reliance on unidimensional models in the conceptualization, assessment, and treatment of depressive disorders. This conceptual deficit is true of the field as a whole (Mann 1988) but is even more evident in studies of depression and other psychiatric disorders in African-Americans and other ethnic groups (Fabrega et al. 1988). Recent evidence implicating biological factors in the etiology of depression (especially the more chronic, severe depressive illnesses) and the evidence implicating psychological, social, and cognitive factors in vulnerability to depression are especially worth noting. Unfortunately, however, few if any studies address these issues in African-Americans, either separately or concurrently. The one exception to this statement is the growing interest in the possibility that there may be biological differences between African-Americans, Caucasians, and other racial and ethnic groups that might explain some of the observed ethnic differences in response to psychoactive agents (Raskin and Crook 1975; Strickland et al. 1991). However, considerations such as inadequacies in the study samples; failure to control for social class, gender, age, and chronicity of illness; questions about the accuracy of diagnostic decisions; and failure to consider nonbiological factors in investigating these hypothesized racial differences in treatment response limit the validity and clinical utility of any conclusions that can be drawn from the available evidence.

PROPOSED BIOPSYCHOSOCIAL MODEL OF DEPRESSION IN AFRICAN-AMERICANS

In this chapter, I argue for the need to move away from unidimensional, ethnic comparison studies of depressive disorders and toward studies focused specifically on within-group differences in vulnerability and treatment response. I also present a case for the need to use more integrative, multidimensional biopsychosocial model of this disorder. Such a model defines depressive disorders as the product of the interaction of both biological (e.g., biochemical dysregulation) and psychosocial factors (e.g., life stresses, dysfunctional cognitions, and interpersonal processes) that moderate risk in people who are at high biopsychosocial risk for this disorder.

Unipolar depression is a complex and heterogeneous clinical syndrome in its own right, independent of the complexities that arise by introducing issues of ethnicity, social class, and gender (Beckham and Leber 1985). Therefore, the proposed conceptual model recommends careful specification of the subgroup of depressive disorders studied. Thus, for example, the significance of the factors studied may vary if we investigate their contributions in predicting symptoms of psychological distress and dysphoria (Kessler et al. 1985) versus their contributions in predicting the onset and course of signs and symptoms in clinical depression (e.g., dysthymia, major depressive disorder; Brown et al. 1987).

Finally, I include consideration of cofactors such as essential hypertension and its risk factors (e.g., obesity, sodium handling, cardiovascular reactivity) because of their potential contribution to vulnerability to depression in African-Americans or their potential to confound results in studies of depression in this population.

Endocrine and Hemodynamic Dysregulation in Depression

Current evidence implicates the dysregulation of norepinephrine, cortisol, dopamine, serotonin (5-HT), and methoxyhydroxyphenylglycol (MHPG) as part of a biological vulnerability to major depressive illness, especially to chronic endogenous depression (Ballenger 1988; McNeal and Cimbolic 1986; Siever and

Davis 1985; Thase and Howland 1989; Thase et al. 1985). Both evidence of amine depletions and amine excesses (norepinephrine and dopamine; Lake et al. 1982) have been reported, as well as both hypersecretion and hyposecretion of cortisol in depression (Ballenger 1988; Thase and Howland 1989). However, whether such dysregulations are the causes or consequences of depression remains unclear. What seems evident, as concluded by Siever and Davis (1985), is that depression results from the dysregulation of the neurotransmitter and endocrine homeostatic regulatory mechanisms and that the different patterns of biochemical dysregulation underscore the biological heterogeneity of depression.

Although research on the various biochemical dysregulation hypotheses has been increasing, comparatively less attention has been given to psychophysiologic parameters. Most such studies have focused on differences between depressed and nondepressed subjects on electrophysiologic parameters (e.g., electroencephalogram, symptom checklist), with little attention paid to hemodynamic parameters. The exception to this rule includes a few studies that investigated the effects of TCAs on blood pressure and heart rate (Goodwin et al. 1978), hemodynamic changes in depressed patients in response to the stress of lumbar puncture (Braier et al. 1988), and one study that used a laboratory stressor (the cold pressor test) to investigate plasma norepinephrine differences between depressed patients and control subjects (Roy et al. 1987). This limited attention to hemodynamic mechanisms is somewhat surprising given the role catecholamines play in cardiovascular reactivity to stress (Houston 1986).

Unfortunately—and regardless of whether we review studies of biochemical, electrophysiologic, or hemodynamic parameters—few if any studies of biological factors in depression included African-Americans or considered whether the patterns of hemodynamic and endocrine dysregulations observed were consistent across ethnic or racial groups. This is an important lacuna in our knowledge, because it is possible that some of the reported ethnic differences in response to antidepressant and antimanic medications (e.g., differences in dose-response curves, differences in risk for side effects; Strickland et al. 1991) might be associated with different patterns of physiological dysregulation in depressed African-American subjects.

It would also be instructive to know whether the hypothesized pattern of biologic dysregulation observed in patients with major depressive disorder is generic to all forms of depression (i.e., depressogenic diathesis) or whether there are distinct dysregulatory patterns for each subtype of depressive disorder. Factors such as age, gender, SES, number of previous episodes, severity of current and previous disorder, types of psychotropic and other medications used, health history and current physical health, and history of substance use and abuse must all be carefully assessed.

BIOBEHAVIORAL REACTIVITY TO STRESS

It is worth noting that research on the biochemical and physiologic dysregulations in depression could be significantly enhanced if investigators would recognize and utilize the techniques of biobehavioral stress reactivity that have proved so useful in research on cardiovascular diseases and hypertension. In an effort to identify the biobehavioral mechanisms that are hypothesized to be dysregulated in hypertension (Schwartz et al. 1979), researchers in cardiovascular behavioral medicine developed and refined a variety of experimental strategies for testing the effect of stressors in the laboratory and under ambulatory conditions. The basic procedure involves exposing subjects who differ in blood pressure status (e.g., hypertensive subjects versus normotensive control subjects), in level of risk for hypertension (e.g., those with and without a family history of hypertension), or subtypes of hypertensive patients (e.g., low- versus high-renin hypertensive subjects) to a variety of psychological, physical, or pharmacologic stressors and measuring the magnitude of change from baseline in a variety of hemodynamic and endocrine parameters (see Schneiderman et al. 1989 for a detailed description.)

This methodology has proven useful in exploring African-American–Caucasian differences in cardiovascular physiology (Anderson 1989) and would be an inexpensive and efficient way of investigating different patterns of biochemical dysregulation in response to defined stressors among various groups of depressed patients.

HYPERTENSION AND RELATED COFACTORS IN DEPRESSION IN AFRICAN-AMERICANS

The extensive epidemiologic and clinical evidence indicating the high prevalence of essential hypertension among African-Americans is an important consideration for research on depression in this population. There is also a growing body of evidence suggesting that the disproportionate burden of risk for hypertension in African-Americans is attributable in part to differences in kidney function, especially in sodium management (Blaustein and Grim 1991) and to differences in hemodynamic and neuroendocrine reactivity to stress (Anderson 1989). Because many of the mechanisms involved in blood pressure control are also implicated in the management of mood, there is reason to suspect that there may also be African-American–Caucasian differences in the biological mechanism implicated in depressive disorders.

For example, research on hypertension indicates that, compared to Caucasians, African-Americans evidence a tendency to conserve sodium and a deficiency in sodium excretion. Grim and colleagues (Grim and Wilson 1989; Grim et al. 1984) have hypothesized that this is a genetically determined trait that had survival benefits in West Africa, where salt was scarce. However, in our modern society where salt is abundant, a salt-conserving trait is no longer health-enhancing. Instead, a low sodium excretion trait and low dietary intake of calcium, potassium, and magnesium combine to increase the risk in African-Americans to a volume-dependent type of hypertension (Blaustein and Grim 1991). In a comprehensive review of the literature on hypertension in African-Americans, Anderson (1989) noted that the tendency toward sodium conservation has been associated with cardiovascular hyperreactivity to stress in the laboratory (Dimsdale et al. 1987; Light et al. 1983). This tendency has been demonstrated in healthy, low-risk normotensive subjects, in healthy normotensive subjects with a family history of hypertension, and in African-American versus Caucasian hypertensive subjects.

The greater vulnerability to hypertension in African-Americans is associated with a host of cofactors, such as obesity, alcohol consumption, low SES, high-fat diets, and so on, all of which must be taken into consideration in studies testing biochemical dysregulation hypotheses in depression in African-Americans.

Relevant to our interest in biochemical and hemodynamic dysregulation in depression is the growing evidence that African-Americans show greater cardiovascular reactivity to stressors that trigger more alpha-adrenergically mediated response systems. These responses are characterized by blood pressure increases resulting from increases in norepinephrine and in total peripheral resistance and slower diastolic blood pressure recovery, but little or no increase in heart rate (Anderson et al. 1991).

Taken as a whole, this evidence therefore suggests that more studies are needed to investigate whether depressed African-American subjects evidence similar or different patterns of electrophysiologic, neuroendocrine, and hemodynamic dysregulation compared to depressed Caucasian subjects. Such studies must pay particular attention to the potential confounding role that obesity, diet, blood pressure, and related factors might have on their findings.

PSYCHOSOCIAL FACTORS IN DEPRESSION

There is a substantial body of empirical evidence, largely independent of the evidence of biological vulnerability, that a host of psychosocial factors also play a major role in conferring risk for depression. These factors have been shown to contribute to vulnerability to depression (Brown and Harris 1978; Paykel 1979, 1982) and to affect the timing of onset and the severity of depressive symptoms (Brown et al. 1987).

These psychosocial risk factors operate largely in three domains: personal, situational, and familial (Hammen 1990). For example, there is substantial consensus that stressful life experiences such as loss of employment or loss of a spouse or significant other increases risk for depression. Thus, events that are negative, uncontrollable, and unexpected and that involve losses or exits are particularly depressogenic (Finlay-Jones and Brown 1981; Paykel 1979). However, the likelihood that such negative life events will result in clinical depression increases as a function of the severity of the events (Brown et al. 1987) and of the presence of preexisting interpersonal vulnerabilities such as the absence of intimate, supportive social attachments (Brown and Harris 1978; Oatley and Bolton 1985).

The depressogenic potential of negative life experiences is also enhanced by early childhood experiences, such as early loss of parents (Brown et al. 1987), early psychosocial deprivation, dysfunctional family relationships, and chronic stresses resulting from maternal depression (Hammen et al. 1987a, 1987b), as well as by negative self- and situational schemata that reinforce feelings of helplessness, hopelessness, and low self-worth (Beck 1987; Beck et al. 1983; Hammen 1988). The evidence is accumulating that these personal, situational, and familial risk factors interact to create a psychosocial diathesis that confers the greatest risk to those who possess more of these psychosocial vulnerabilities.

Thus far I have considered the evidence of vulnerability conferred by factors proximal to the individual. However, this analysis would be incomplete if it failed to consider vulnerability factors in the distal context (i.e., the community at large). Factors such as chronic poverty and ethnic and gender-role oppression should also be considered as potentially depressogenic, because they limit life opportunities and reinforce feelings of hopelessness and low perceived control over life circumstances. However, it should be noted that these broad contextual factors confer risk at the macro level. Their role in predicting individual risk for clinical depression is mediated by those personal, contextual, and familial attributes discussed previously.

PSYCHOSOCIAL RISK FACTORS AND DEPRESSION IN AFRICAN-AMERICANS

Although evidence in support of the contribution of psychosocial factors in depression has continued to grow, very little research has been conducted to test these hypothesized relationships in African-Americans. There is little reason to expect that negative life events, chronic life stresses, early psychosocial deprivation and dysfunctional family relationships that are a consequence of maternal depression, the absence of intimate, supportive social attachments, or negative self and situational schemata should be any less depressogenic in African-Americans than in Caucasians or any other group. However, because the social conditions of African-Americans in society are so different from those of Caucasians, it is possible that these psychosocial risk factors for depression may operate differently.

For example, despite the heavier burden of socioeconomic deprivation experienced by African-Americans, evidence from the Epidemiologic Catchment Area (ECA) studies did not confirm expectations that there would be a greater prevalence of depressive disorders in African-Americans than in Caucasians (Robins 1991). This was true whether lifetime or current prevalence of major depression was assessed (Charney and Weissman 1988; Robins 1991) or whether subtypes of depression were considered (Weissman et al. 1991). However, studies of depressed patients in treatment consistently note differences in treatment settings, in social status, and in pattern of symptomatology (Fabrega et al. 1988). These differences suggest that various factors may be implicated or that the same risk factors may be interacting differently to confer vulnerability to or protection from depressive disorders in African-Americans and Caucasians. In the absence of empirical tests of these hypotheses, we can only speculate about such possibilities.

In sum, there is some evidence that African-Americans may evidence different patterns of symptoms of depression than Caucasians do, although it is not clear whether the differences observed are real or an artifact of diagnostic errors or whether they result from the high comorbidity from substance use and other disorders that may be more prevalent among African-Americans. There is somewhat better evidence suggesting African-American–Caucasian differences in response to psychotropic agents, which may indicate different underlying biological processes in at least some subgroups of depressed African-American subjects. Unfortunately, little research has been conducted on the contributions of psychosocial factors in conferring risk for depression in African-Americans.

Nevertheless, there is substantial justification and need for carefully designed studies that give specific attention to testing the major biochemical dysregulation and psychosocial vulnerability hypotheses in African-Americans. Considerable care must be exercised in the selection of study samples, paying particular attention to demographics, life-style, and health history. Also, because of the ongoing debate about the appropriateness of current assessment and diagnostic methods, investigators are advised to be especially sensitive to potential sources of diagnostic biases and errors. These methodological concerns can be addressed by not relying solely on self-report measures of depression, but by using carefully trained, experienced interviewers and the best structured diagnostic interview protocols currently available (e.g., the Structured Clinical Interview for DSM-III-R [SCID; Spitzer and Williams 1985], Diagnostic Interview Schedule [DIS; Robins et al. 1981], Schedule for Affective Disorders and Schizophrenia, Lifetime Version [SADS-L; Endicott and Spitzer 1978], etc.) in their subject ascertainment. The former can be very useful in exploring differences in symptom expression but are inadequate if used alone in clinical studies. By the same token, structured interviews are most useful when interviewers are specifically trained and experienced in working with African-American patients. Also, the conventional wisdom that indicates that better and more reliable conclusions can be drawn from studies that focus on specific clinical subgroups applies here.

Finally—and consistent with a biopsychosocial perspective on depression—it is our contention that the best and most useful studies of these disorders in African-Americans will be those that investigate the interplay between psychosocial and biological factors. For example, our understanding of depressive disorders in African-Americans and the treatment of such disorders would be significantly enhanced by studies that investigate whether chronic life stresses and life events trigger endocrine dysregulation in African-Americans at risk for depression (e.g., those with a personal or maternal history of depression), and whether these endocrine effects are associated with pattern and severity of symptoms, course of illness, treatment response and treatment outcome, and risk for relapse. Similarly, studies of the differential effects of antidepressants would be greatly improved if life stresses and personality characteristics were taken into consideration as possible sources of variance in treatment response.

In this chapter, I have reviewed and discussed the limited evidence available on biopsychosocial factors implicated in depression in African-Americans. Our understanding and the effectiveness of our efforts to treat these disorders in this population are limited by the lack of empirical research. I hope that this chapter will stimulate and encourage researchers to pursue some of the exciting theoretical and clinical questions raised.

REFERENCES

Abramson LY, Seligman M, Teasdale JD: Learned helplessness: critique and reformulation. J Abnorm Psychol 87:49–74, 1978

Adebimpe VE: Overview: white norms and psychiatric diagnosis of black patients. Am J Psychiatry 138:279–285, 1981

Adebimpe VR, Gigandet J, Harris E: MMPI diagnosis of black psychiatric patients. Am J Psychiatry 136:85–87, 1979

Adebimpe VR, Hedlund JL, Cho DW, et al: Symptomatology of depression in black and white patients. J Natl Med Assoc 74:185–190, 1982

Anderson NB: Ethnic differences in resting and stress-induced cardiovascular and humoral activity: an overview, in Handbook of Research Methods in Cardiovascular Behavioral Medicine. Edited by Schneiderman N, Weiss SB, Kaufman PG. New York, Plenum, 1989, pp 433–452

Anderson NB, McNeilly M, Myers HF: Autonomic reactivity and hypertension in blacks: a review and proposed model. Ethnicity and Disease 1:154–170, 1991

Ballenger JC: Biological aspects of depression: implications for clinical practice, in American Psychiatric Press Review of Psychiatry, Vol 7. Edited by Frances AJ, Hales RE. Washington, DC, American Psychiatric Press, 1988, pp 169–187

Baskin D, Bluestone H, Nelson M: Mental illness in minority women. J Clin Psychol 37:491–498, 1981

Beck AT: Cognitive models of depression. Journal of Cognitive Psychotherapy: An International Quarterly 1:5–37, 1987

Beck AT, Epstein N, Harrison R: Cognitions, attitudes and personality dimensions in depression. British Journal of Cognitive Psychotherapy 1:1–16, 1983

Beckham EE, Leber WR (eds): Handbook of Depression: Treatment, Assessment and Research. Homewood, IL, Dorsey Press, 1985

Blaustein MP, Grim CE: The pathogenesis of hypertension: Black-White differences, in Cardiovascular Diseases in Blacks. Edited by Saunders E. Philadelphia, PA, FA Davis & Co, 1991, pp 97–114

Braier A, Wolkowitz, OM, Doran AR, et al: Neurobiological effects of lumbar puncture stress in psychiatric patients and healthy volunteers. Psychiatry Res 25:187–194, 1988

Brown GW, Harris T: Social Origins of Depression. London, Tavistock, 1978

Brown GW, Bifulco A, Harris TO: Life events, vulnerability and onset of depression. Br J Psychiatry 150:30–42, 1987

Bureau of the Census: 1990 Census: Age, Sex, and Race for the United States, Regions and States. Washington, DC, U.S. Department of Commerce, 1990

Charney EA, Weissman MM: Epidemiology of depressive illness, in Phenomenology of Depressive Illness. Edited by Mann JJ. New York, Human Sciences Press, 1988, pp 45–74

Cheung FK: Minority population use of mental health services in the community, in Ethnic Minority Perspectives on Clinical Training and Services in Psychology. Edited by Myers H, Wolhford P, Guzman LP, et al. Washington, DC, American Psychological Association, 1991, pp 23–32

Cheung FK, Snowden LR: Community mental health and ethnic minority populations. Community Ment Health J 26:277–291, 1990

Cooper RS: A note on the biological concept of race and its application in epidemiologic research. Am Heart J 108:715–723, 1984

Cooper RS: Celebrate diversity—or should we? Ethnicity and Disease 1:3–7, 1991

Crews DE, Bindon JR: Ethnicity as a taxonomic category in biomedical and biosocial research. Ethnicity and Disease 1:424–449, 1991

Derogatis L, Lipman R, Covi L, et al: Neurotic symptom dimensions: as perceived by psychiatrists and patients of various social classes. Arch Gen Psychiatry 24:455–464, 1971

Dimsdale JE, Graham RM, Ziegler MG, et al: Age, race, diagnosis and sodium effects on the pressor response to infused norepinephrine. Hypertension 10:564–569, 1987

Dressler WW: Unemployment and depressive symptoms in a southern black community. J Nerv Ment Dis 174:639–645, 1986

Dressler WW, Badger LW: Epidemiology of depressive symptoms in black communities: a comparative analysis. J Nerv Ment Dis 173:212–220, 1985

Edwards A: The consequences of error in selecting treatments for blacks. Social Casework: The Journal of Contemporary Social Work 63:429–433, 1982

Endicott J, Spitzer RL: A diagnostic interview: the Schedule for Affective Disorders and Schizophrenia. Arch Gen Psychiatry 35:837–844, 1978

Fabrega H, Mezzich J, Ulrich RF: Black-White differences in psychopathology in an urban psychiatric population. Compr Psychiatry 29:285–297, 1988

Fellini P: Perspectives on depression among Black Americans. Health Soc Work 14:245–252, 1989

Finlay-Jones R, Brown GW: Types of stressful life events and the onset of anxiety and depressive disorders. Psychol Med 11:803–815, 1981

Galanter M, Castaneda R, Ferman J: Substance abuse among general psychiatric patients: place of presentation, diagnosis and treatment. Am J Drug Alcohol Abuse 14:211–235, 1988

Goodwin FK, Cowdry RW, Webster MK: Predictors of drug response in the affective disorders: toward an integrated approach, in Psychopharmacology: A Generation of Progress. Edited by Lipton MA, DiMascio A, Killam KF. New York, Raven, 1978, pp 1277–1288

Gould SJ: The Mismeasure of Man. New York, WW Norton, 1981

Grim CE, Wilson TW: The worldwide epidemiology of hypertension in blacks with a note on a new theory for the greater prevalence of hypertension in Western Hemisphere blacks, in Hypertension in Black and Other Minorities: 1988 Conference Proceedings of the Second Annual Nutrition Workshop. Edited by Enuonwee CO. Nashville, TN, Meharry Medical College, 1989, pp 57–73

Grim CE, Luft FC, Weinberg MH, et al: Genetic, familial and racial influences on blood pressure control systems in man. Aust N Z J Med 14:453–457, 1984

Hammen C: Depression and cognitions about stressful life events, in Cognitive Processes in Depression. Edited by Alloy L. New York, Guilford, 1988, pp 77–108

Hammen C: Vulnerability to depression: personal, situational, and family aspects, in Contemporary Approaches to Depression: Treatment, Research, and Theory. Edited by Ingram R. New York, Plenum, 1990, pp 59–69

Hammen C, Gordon D, Burge D, et al: Maternal affective disorders, illness and stress: risk for children's psychopathology. Am J Psychiatry 144:736–741, 1987a

Hammen C, Gordon D, Burge D, et al: Communication patterns of mothers with affective disorders and their relationship to children's status and social functioning, in Understanding Major Mental Disorders: The Contribution of Family Interaction Research. Edited by Hahlberg K, Goldstein M. New York, Family Process Press, 1987b, pp 103–119

Hanson B, Klerman GL: Interracial problems in the assessment of clinical depression: concordance differences between white psychiatrists and black and white patients. Psychopharmacol Bull 10:65–66, 1974

Heizer J: Bipolar affective disorders in black and white men: a comparison of symptoms and familial illness. Arch Gen Psychiatry 32:1140–1143, 1975

Houston BK: Psychological variables and cardiovascular and neuroendocrine reactivity, in Handbook of Stress, Reactivity and Cardiovascular Disease. Edited by Mathews K, Weiss SM, Detre T, et al. New York, Wiley, 1986, pp 207–229

Kessler RC, Neighbors HW: A new perspective on the relationships among race, social class and psychological distress. J Health Soc Behav 27:107–115, 1986

Kessler RC, Price RH, Wortman CB: Social factors in psychopathology: stress, social support and coping processes. Annu Rev Psychol 36:531–572, 1985

Lake CR, Pickar D, Ziegler MG, et al: High plasma norepinephrine levels in patients with major affective disorder. Am J Psychiatry 139:1315–1318, 1982

Lawson WB: Racial and ethnic factors in psychiatric research. Hosp Community Psychiatry 37:50–54, 1986

Light KC, Koepke JP, Obrist PA, et al: Psychological stress induces sodium and fluid retention in men at high risk for hypertension. Science 220:429–431, 1983

Lin KM, Poland RE, Lesser IM: Ethnicity and psychopharmacology. Cult Med Psychiatry 10:151–165, 1986

Mann JJ (ed): Phenomenology of Depressive Illness. New York, Human Sciences Press, 1988

McNeal E, Cimbolic P: Antidepressants and biochemical theories of depression. Psychol Bull 99:361–374, 1986

Montagu A: Man's Most Dangerous Myth: The Fallacy of Race. New York, Columbia University Press, 1945

Neighbors HW, Jackson JS, Campbell L, et al: The influence of racial factors on psychiatric diagnosis: a review and suggestions for research. Community Ment Health J 25:301–311, 1989

Oatley K, Bolton W: A social-cognitive theory of depression in reaction to life events. Psychol Rev 92:372–388, 1985

Paykel ES: Causal relationships between clinical depression and life events, in Stress and Mental Disorder. Edited by Barrett J, Rose R, Klerman G. New York, Raven, 1979, pp 71–86

Paykel ES: Life events and early environment, in Handbook of Affective Disorders. Edited by Paykel ES. Edinburgh, Scotland, Churchill-Livingstone Press, 1982, pp 146–161

President's Commission on Mental Health: Report to the President. Washington, DC, U.S. Government Printing Office, 1978

Raskin A, Crook TH: Antidepressants in black and white inpatients. Arch Gen Psychiatry 32:643–649, 1975

Raskin A, Crook TH, Herman KD: Psychiatric history and symptom differences in black and white depressed patients. J Consult Clin Psychol 43:73–80, 1975

Richards JM, Gottfredson GD: Health status of minorities and low income groups (DHHS Publ No HRS-P-DV85-1). Washington, DC, U.S. Government Printing Office, 1985

Robins LN: An overview of psychiatric disorders in America, in Psychiatric Disorders in America: The Epidemiologic Catchment Area Study. Edited by Robins LN, Regier DA. New York, Free Press, 1991, pp 328–566

Robins LN, Helzer JE, Croughan J, et al: National Institute of Mental Health Diagnostic Interview Schedule: its history, characteristics, and validity. Arch Gen Psychiatry 38:381–389, 1981

Robins LN, Helzer JE, Weissman MM, et al: Lifetime prevalence of specific psychiatric disorders in three sites. Arch Gen Psychiatry 41:941–958, 1984

Roy A, Guthrie S, Pickar D, et al: Plasma norepinephrine responses to cold challenge in depressed patients and normal controls. Psychiatric Review 21:161–168, 1987

Schneiderman N, Weiss SB, Kaufman PG: Handbook of Research Methods in Cardiovascular Behavioral Medicine. New York, Plenum, 1989

Schwartz GE, Shapiro AP, Redmond DP, et al: Behavioral medicine approaches to hypertension: an integrative analysis of theory and research. J Behav Med 2:11–364, 1979

Siever LJ, Davis KL: Overview: toward a dysregulation hypothesis of depression. Am J Psychiatry 142:1017–1031, 1985

Simon J, Fleiss JE, Gurland BJ, et al: Depression and schizophrenia in hospitalized black and white mental patients. Arch Gen Psychiatry 28:509–512, 1973

Somervell PP, Leaf PJ, Weissman MM, et al: The prevalence of major depression in black and white adults in five United States communities. Am J Epidemiol 130:725–735, 1989

Spitzer RL, Williams T: Structured Clinical Interview for DSM-III-R Personality Disorders. New York, Biometrics Research Department of New York State Psychiatric Institute, 1985

Strickland TL, Ranganath V, Lin KM, et al: Psychopharmacologic considerations in the treatment of black American populations. Psychopharmacol Bull 27:441–448, 1991

Sue S: Psychotherapeutic services for ethnic minorities: some optimism, some pessimism. Am Psychol 43:301–308, 1988

Taube CA, Barrett SA (eds): Mental health in the United States (DHHS Publ No ADM-85-1378). Rockville, MD, U.S. Government Printing Office, 1985

Thase ME, Howland R: The biology of depression. Paper presented at the Boulder Symposium in Clinical Psychology: Depression, Boulder, CO, April 1989

Thase ME, Frank E, Kupfer DJ: Biological processes in major depression, in Handbook of Depression: Treatment, Assessment and Research. Edited by Beckham EE, Leber WR. Homewood, IL, Dorsey Press, 1985, pp 816–913

Tonks C, Paykel ES, Klerman GL: Clinical depression among Negroes. Am J Psychiatry 127:327–335, 1970

Uhlenhuth E, Paykel E: Symptom configuration and life events. Arch Gen Psychiatry 28:747–748, 1973

Warheit G, Holzer C, Schwab J: An analysis of social class and racial differences in depressive symptomatology: a community study. J Health Soc Behav 14:291–299, 1973

Warheit G, Holzer CE, Schwab JJ: An analysis of social class and racial differences in depressive symptomatology: a community sample. J Health Soc Behav 14:291–299, 1987

Weissman MM, Leaf PJ, Bruce ML, et al: The epidemiology of dysthymia in five communities: rates, risks, comorbidity and treatment. Am J Psychiatry 145:815–819, 1988

Weissman MM, Bruce ML, Leaf PJ, et al: Affective disorders, in Psychiatric Disorders in America: The Epidemiologic Catchment Area Study. Edited by Robins LN, Regier DA. New York, Free Press, 1991, pp 53–80

Williams DH: The epidemiology of mental illness in Afro-Americans. Hosp Community Psychiatry 37:42–49, 1986

Wood AJ, Zhou HH: Ethnic differences in drug disposition and responsiveness. Clin Pharmacol 20:1–24, 1991

Ziegler VE, Biggs JT: Tricyclic plasma levels. JAMA 14:2167–2169, 1977

Zung WW, MacDonald J, Zung E: Prevalence of clinically significant depressive symptoms in black and white patients in family practice settings. Am J Psychiatry 145:882–883, 1988

Chapter 13

Clinical and Epidemiologic Studies of Dementias: Cross-Ethnic Perspectives

Linda Chang, M.S., M.D.,
Bruce L. Miller, M.D., and
Keh-Ming Lin, M.D., M.P.H.

There are a multitude of medical diseases that can cause dementia, and cross-cultural epidemiological studies into many of the dementing conditions are still greatly needed. The etiology for most of the dementias is unknown, although the Guamanian dementia syndromes and prion-related diseases are two examples of how cross-cultural studies can offer important clues into potential causes and preventions for dementing illnesses.

In this chapter the prevalence and costs for the various dementing conditions are outlined. This is followed by a brief discussion of some of the unique problems associated with performing cross-cultural research into dementia—particularly the difficulty in obtaining an accurate diagnosis. Next there is a discussion of the cross-cultural studies that have been performed with specific dementias that include: Alzheimer's disease (AD), vascular dementia, frontal lobe degeneration (FLD), parkinsonian dementia, the Guamanian-amyotrophic lateral sclerosis/parkinsonian (ALS/PD) dementia syndrome, prion diseases (*kuru*, Creutzfeldt-Jakob disease [CJD], and Gerstmann-Straussler syndrome), and acquired immunodeficiency syn-

---

Supported in part by a grant from the National Institute of Aging to the UCLA Alzheimer Center (AG10123) and the National Institute of Mental Health Research Center on the Psychobiology of Ethnicity (MH47193).

drome (AIDS) dementia. Finally, future directions in research are suggested.

PREVALENCE AND COSTS

The commonest and most costly dementia syndrome worldwide is AD. Recent estimates indicate that AD is the fourth leading cause of death in the United States, ranking behind only heart disease, cancer, and stroke (Vinters et al. 1988). There is an estimated prevalence of 4 million (Evans et al. 1989) for AD, with somewhere between 100,000 and 200,000 deaths per year. The costs associated with AD are staggering; Hay and Ernst (1987) estimated that the cost of care for patients with AD was in the range of $27 billion to $100 billion annually. Figures for other dementing conditions are less certain, although vascular-, parkinsonian-, and AIDS-dementia syndromes all account for serious morbidity and mortality. Both AD and AIDS dementia will be increasing in the coming years, and there is little likelihood that either will be curable in the foreseeable future.

With AD, no preventable or reversible factor has been discovered. The only two well-established risk factors for AD are genetics and aging—neither of which can be altered. Vascular dementia is the second most common cause for dementia, and many risk factors have been defined for this disease (Liu et al. 1992). As we will discuss, there appear to be significant differences in prevalence rates for AD and vascular dementia (as well as many of the other dementing conditions) among Caucasians, blacks, and Asians (de la Monte et al. 1989; Shibayama et al. 1986). Although some of this variation is probably due purely to different patterns of diagnosis, real differences in prevalence appear to exist.

Similarly, FLDs (Miller et al. 1991) have no known reversible or treatable risk factors, and there may be worldwide variations in this condition. Parkinson's disease (PD) appears to have regional variations in prevalence (Schoenberg 1987; Schoenberg et al. 1987), although there are few well-known etiologic factors (as we discuss later in this chapter). With many of these conditions, cross-cultural studies may provide important clues about potential genetic and environmental risk factors.

ACCURACY OF DIAGNOSIS FOR DEMENTING CONDITIONS

One confounding feature of research into dementing conditions is that diagnosis during a patient's life is significantly flawed for all dementia syndromes. Recent attempts to formalize research criteria for AD have greatly improved diagnostic accuracy (McKhann et al. 1984). However, despite significant improvement in the diagnosis of AD over the past two decades, even at the best research centers in the United States, 10%–27% of patients dying with a diagnosis of AD are found to have had a different disease at the time of death (Boller et al. 1989; Joachim et al. 1988). Outside of research centers, diagnostic accuracy is undoubtedly far worse. As we will see, many of the previously performed cross-cultural studies into dementia have had flawed methods for diagnosis, and this has limited the value of these studies.

For other dementing conditions, diagnostic accuracy is even worse than with AD. For example, in a study of 11 patients diagnosed as having a mixed dementia secondary to AD and multiple strokes, 5 had autopsy confirmation of a mixed dementia, 3 had AD, 2 had multi-infarct dementia, and 1 had multiple sclerosis (Thal et al. 1991). Although no definitive figures are available for the FLDs and parkinsonian-dementia syndromes, with both conditions misdiagnosis is high (Thal et al. 1991). In fact, even with simple PD, clinical diagnoses are often flawed—in one study of patients with a diagnosis of PD, pathological confirmation was found in only 76% of the patients (Rajput et al. 1991).

In contrast, diagnosis of the Guamanian-ALS/PD dementias and AIDS dementia is remarkably accurate. With the Guamanian-ALS/PD dementia syndrome, diagnosis is accurate, because this distinctive clinical syndrome is the main cause for dementia in Guam. With AIDS dementia, diagnosis is good because an accurate serologic test exists.

One way to improve diagnosis in cross-cultural epidemiological studies would be to insist that patients' clinical diagnosis be confirmed with a postmortem examination. Although clinical studies lack accuracy, sole reliance on pathological studies is also flawed. Does a patient with pathological findings of AD who is not demented have AD? Similarly, it is unclear if those who were without signs of PD during life but who, in postmortem examinations, reveal changes in the brain typical of the disease should be regarded as truly having had this illness.

CROSS-CULTURAL DEMENTIA STUDIES: GENERAL CONCERNS

Perhaps the greatest problem with epidemiological cross-cultural research into dementia has been that the methods for diagnosis have differed from study to study. For example, some epidemiological studies have utilized loose clinical criteria for diagnosing the dementia; in many instances, neuropsychological tests have not been included in the determination of dementia type. Additionally, in several studies, the determination of the cause for the dementia was made by neurological and psychiatric specialists (Li et al. 1989; Shibayama et al. 1986; Zhang et al. 1990), whereas others made diagnoses based on interviews made by nonmedical personnel (Copeland et al. 1987).

In many of the cross-cultural studies performed, the age or educational levels of the selected population have significantly differed from the general population. As a result, findings derived from these studies did not necessarily reflect the prevalence of that disease in the whole population. Examples can be seen in studies that have evaluated only nursing home patients (Serby et al. 1987) or patients referred through postal surveys (Garland 1952). In future epidemiological studies, it will be important to select representative populations before broad generalizations can be made regarding the prevalence of a disease.

Compounding these problems, tools that are used to quantify dementia in one country may not be valid elsewhere. One study that illustrated this problem compared performance on the Mini-Mental Status Exam (MMSE; Folstein et al. 1975) in Finland and China (Salmon et al. 1989). The MMSE is a standard scale that is used to quantify dementia in the United States; to meet a research diagnosis of AD, a subject must score below 25 on the MMSE. In a study by Salmon and colleagues (1989), it was found that education greatly influenced MMSE scores. The Finnish and Chinese groups had similar scores when the education variable was controlled for. The Finnish group performed better on orientation to time, registration of three objects, obeying a three-step command, reading a sentence, and copying a pentagon. In contrast, the Shanghai subjects tested better on serial 7s, recall of three objects, and repetition of a phrase. These differences probably reflect educational experiences but could influence the prevalence of the diagnosis for dementia.

PREVALENCE OF DEMENTIA IN VARIOUS POPULATIONS

Earlier studies performed in the 1950s and 1960s used the general term "organic brain syndrome" to differentiate dementia from psychiatric illnesses. These studies were performed in surveys of "mental illnesses," and specific dementia syndromes were not described. Although some of these early studies were important steps in defining the prevalence of dementia, they lacked the diagnostic precision of more recent studies, which elucidated a clearer idea for the distribution of specific dementia syndromes. Despite recent advances in diagnoses, many studies continue to report prevalence of dementia only in terms of mild, moderate, or severe, based primarily on performance on clinical examinations or the MMSE or Geriatric MMSE.

Table 13–1 shows the prevalence of dementia in different geographical regions and illustrates that the prevalence of dementia worldwide has ranged from 0.5% to 11.3%. One probable explanation for these differences in prevalence has been that some of these studies included the "mild" and "moderate" dementia subjects, whereas others reported only "severe" cases. Therefore, it is difficult to compare one report with another and to draw meaningful conclusions regarding the differences between the incidence of dementia in these countries. Identical methods for evaluations as well as representative populations from each region are needed in cross-cultural studies.

In the following subsections, we will describe the major dementia syndromes for which some data are available.

Table 13–1. Prevalence of dementia in different geographical regions

Region	Authors (year)	Age surveyed	Number surveyed	Prevalence (%)	Diagnostic method
China					
Shanghai	Zhang et al. 1990	55	5,055	4.6	Clinical, MMSE
Beijing	Li et al. 1989	60+/65+	1,331	1.3/1.8	Clinical, MMSE < 17
Taiwan	Lin 1953	60+	1,113	0.5	Clinical
Singapore	Kua 1991	65	612	1.8	Clinical, GMS(S)***
United States					
Baltimore, MD	de la Monte et al. 1989	24–95	6,000	4.0	Autopsies
Copiah, MS	Schoenberg et al. 1985a	40+/65+	8,925	0.5/2.2	Clinical, MMSE
Rochester, MN	Schoenberg et al. 1987	29+	178*	1.0	Clinical, Pathological[a] every dementia case recorded
Boston, MA	Evans et al. 1989	65+	3,623	10.3	Clinical, Neuropsychological
England					
Newcastle upon Tyne	Kay et al. 1964	65+	297	5.6	Clinical [a]Selected from sample of 1,780
Liverpool	Copeland et al. 1987	65+	1,070	5.2	Clinical, GMS(S)

Sweden	Bollerup 1975	all 70	626	5.0	Clinical
Finland					
Turku	Molsa et al. 1982	65+	520*	2.0	Clinical;[a] selected patients
All areas	Sulkava et al. 1985	30+/65+	8,000	1.8/6.7	Clinical health interview & examinations in selected samples
Japan					
Nagoya	Shibayama et al. 1986	65+	3,106	5.8	Clinical
Tokyo	Karasawa et al. 1982	65+	4,502	4.6	Clinical
Italy					
Appignano	Rocca et al. 1990	59+	778	6.2	Clinical, MMSE
Israel	Treves et al. 1986	40–60	71*	2.4	Clinical

Note. MMSE = Mini-Mental State Exam in Chinese; GMS(S) = Geriatric Mental State Scale.
[a] Neurologic Disease Register.

Alzheimer's Disease

The clinical-pathological syndrome. One problem with cross-cultural studies of AD is that several different terms have been used to describe patients with AD. Various terms—senile dementia of Alzheimer type, senile brain syndrome, primary degenerative dementia, and senile dementia—have been used. The cause of this progressive degenerative disorder is unknown, although patients with AD show characteristic abnormalities on histologic sections of the brain and the clinical course follows a characteristic progression. Pathological studies classically show cerebral atrophy with neuritic (senile) plaques in cerebral cortex and accumulations of neurofibrillary tangles in large pyramidal neurons (Cummings and Benson 1983).

Early clinical signs can be subtle: forgetfulness, intellectual fatigue, diminished language skills, and mood and personality changes (e.g., depression or paranoia). Later, a cortical dementia predominates, with aphasia, memory and cognitive impairment, and relatively preserved motor function (Vinters et al. 1988). Structural imaging modalities such as computed tomography (CT) and magnetic resonance imaging (MRI) demonstrate generalized atrophy in most patients with AD, although neither modality can be reliably used to make a definitive AD diagnosis (Leedom and Miller 1990). More recent advances in functional neuroimaging utilizing positron-emission tomography (PET) and single photon emission computed tomography (SPECT) to evaluate cerebral metabolism and blood flow may improve diagnostic accuracy. Typically, AD patients develop bilateral temporal and parietal hypometabolism (detectable by PET) or hypoperfusion (detectable by SPECT); however, this pattern can sometimes be seen in other diseases (e.g., sleep apnea, posthypoxic dementia, and multi-infarct dementia; Miller et al. 1990).

Epidemiology of AD. Early studies performed in the 1950s and 1960s suggested that dementia was uncommon in Asians and had a higher prevalence among Europeans. For example, in one of the first epidemiological studies performed in Asia, Lin (1953) identified dementia in only 0.5% of elderly subjects over age 60. In comparison, a study performed in England (Kay 1964) showed that 12.2% of the population over age 65 had "organic brain syndrome," and approximately 5% had "senile dementia." These earlier studies not only utilized different methods for diagnosis, but no data were available regarding what percentage of these dementia and organic brain syndromes were because of AD.

More recent studies suggest that AD is the primary cause of dementia in the United States, accounting for 50%–60% of dementia cases among elderly patients and up to 20% in younger patients (Terry and Katzman 1983). In developed countries, most report that AD accounts for approximately one-half of dementia cases (Mortimer 1983). However, studies performed in Asia have reported a much lower prevalence of dementia in general and a lower percentage of AD cases among those diagnosed with dementia (Chen et al. 1987; Shibayama et al. 1986). Some of these differences in prevalence may relate to different patterns in diagnosis rather than true differences in prevalence; in addition, the studies performed in Asian populations have not included postmortem diagnoses.

However, a recent well-designed survey ($N = 5{,}055$) of older Chinese subjects in Shanghai, China, showed that the prevalence rate of dementia in persons 65 years and older was 4.6%, with 65% of this group ($n = 103$) having a clinical diagnosis of AD (Zhang et al. 1990). Prevalence of dementia in the Shanghai study sharply rose from 4.6% among subjects 65 years and older, to 12.3% among those over age 75 and 24.3% among those in the over-85 group. After controlling for cultural and education-dependent variables, the estimate of 65% of the subjects with dementia having a diagnosis of AD was comparable to the prevalence rate of AD for people in developed countries, including Singapore, Japan, the United States, Italy, and Finland (Table 13–2).

The prevalence of AD has been studied among different racial groups in the United States and in other countries. A recent study (de la Monte et al. 1989) from the Johns Hopkins Hospital found, among 6,000 consecutive autopsies, 144 patients had clinical diagnosis of dementia, and 48 had AD. Although the proportions of Caucasians and blacks were similar, the frequency of AD was

Table 13–2. Percentage of diagnosed AD, MID, PD, and other dementias in patients with dementia in different countries

Regions (authors)	AD	MID	PD	Prion diseases	Others[a]
Chinese					
Shanghai, China (Zhang et al. 1990)	64.7	26.8	NS	NS	8.5
Beijing, China (Li et al. 1989)	33.0	61.0	0.0	0.0	6.0
Singapore (Kua 1991)	63.6	36.4	0.0	0.0	none
New York, USA (Serby et al. 1987)	12.1	75.9	4.6	0.0	7.5
Japanese					
Nagoya (Shibayama et al. 1986)	41.4	48.3	Unknown	Unknown	10.3
Tokyo (Karasawa et al. 1982)	18.0	70.0	Unknown	Unknown	12.0
Finnish					
Turku, Finland (Molsa et al. 1982)	51.8	27.6	2.9	0.0	17.7
Finland, all areas (Sulkava et al. 1985)	50.0	39.0	1.4	0.0	11.0
Americans (Caucasian)					
Baltimore, MD (de la Monte et al. 1989)	46.2	5.1	6.4	5.1	37.2
Rochester, MN (Schoenberg et al. 1987)	51.7	5.1	2.8	0.0	40.4
Framingham (Kase et al. 1989)	56.0	9.0	0.0	0.0	35.0
Boston, MA (Evans et al. 1989)	84.1	4.4	0.0	0.0	11.5
Americans (black)					
Baltimore, MD (de la Monte et al. 1989)	18.2	22.7	1.5	0.0	57.6

Table 13–2. Percentage of diagnosed AD, MID, PD, and other dementias in patients with dementia in different countries *(continued)*

Regions (authors)	AD	MID	PD	Prion diseases	Others[a]
British					
Newcastle upon Tyne (Kay et al. 1964)	60.3	29.4	Unknown	Unknown	10.3
Cambridgeshire (rural)[b] (Brayne and Calloway 1989)	52.0	31.0	0.0	0.0	17.0
Italians					
Appignano (Rocca et al. 1990)	42.0	35.0	Unknown	Unknown	23.0

Note. AD = Alzheimer's disease; MID = multi-infarct dementia; NS = not specified; PD = Parkinson's disease.
[a] Others include mixed dementias.
[b] Elderly women ages 70–79.

2.6 times higher among Caucasians ($P = .001$). In Israel, a significantly higher incidence of AD of the presenile type was observed in European- or American-born subjects compared with individuals who were African- or Asian-born (Treves et al. 1986). Several Japanese studies also showed lower incidence of AD in Japan compared with Europe or the United States (Karasawa et al. 1982; Shibayama et al. 1986).

In many studies of AD, there has been a higher prevalence of AD among females than males. This difference could not entirely be explained by the fact that females tend to live longer than males. However, other studies have found no significant differences in prevalence between genders (Fratiglioni et al. 1991; Kohmen et al. 1989), and some actually found a higher prevalence in men (Persson 1980; Pfeffer et al. 1987). In an interesting twist, the Shanghai study (Zhang et al. 1990) showed that females with a lower educational level had a higher prevalence of AD than did females with a higher level of education. Zhang and colleagues hypothesized that the lack of formal education in the elderly female subjects with dementia in China may have been the result of early deprivation and subsequent lower brain reserve, which in turn allowed the clinical symptoms of dementia to appear among these women at a younger age.

Genetic studies in AD. Perhaps the strongest data to suggest that AD has a genetic component have been the work with Down syndrome. Close to 100% of patients with Down syndrome develop the neuropathological changes that are seen in AD (Ellis et al. 1974). More recently, it was reported that some patients with early onset familial AD show an abnormality on chromosome 21 (St. George-Hyslop et al. 1987), further linking the two disorders to a similar genetic mechanism. Another tantalizing clue has been the discovery that there is an increased frequency of dementia secondary to AD or Down syndrome among relatives of patients with nonfamilial AD (Heston et al. 1981). Furthermore, late-onset sporadic familial AD has been associated with chromosome 19 (Schellenberg et al. 1987). In approximately 10% of cases, AD appears to have an autosomal dominant inheritance (Cook et al. 1979; Goudsmit et al. 1981; Nee et al. 1980). However, many cases are sporadic with no clear familial pattern, suggesting a possible environmental influence in determining the development of this disorder. In studies of monozygotic twins, if one twin develops AD, there is a 40%–50% likelihood that the other will develop AD (Heston et al. 1981). However, several studies have shown that the development of AD in the second twin may occur decades later (Cook et al. 1981; Nee et al. 1987). More recent studies also showed discordance of AD in monozygotic twins (Creasey et al. 1989).

In another study (Endo et al. 1986), the genotype of HLA-B16, which occurs at a lower frequency in Japan than in Europe and the United States, was found to be significantly associated with AD. Therefore, the findings support the theory that the difference in prevalence of AD between Japan and other countries is caused by genetic factors. A more recent study also showed a relationship between HLA-A2 and early-onset sporadic AD in men (Payami et al. 1991).

All of these studies support the hypothesis that "sporadic" AD may be genetically determined. Recent linkage studies show genetic heterogeneity in AD, which suggests that AD can be caused by a variety of different mechanisms (St. George-Hyslop et al. 1990; Tanzi et al. 1990). Cross-cultural studies focusing on different genetic makeups will further clarify this issue. These studies in toto strongly suggest that both genetic and environmental factors interact in the pathogenesis of AD. Whether differences in the environment (such as diet) among various cultures may be accountable for the wide range of incidence of AD remains to be shown. However, regional studies will continue to provide important clues for the pathogenesis of AD.

Multi-Infarct Dementia

Clinical characteristics. Progressive cognitive impairment resulting from multiple episodes of cerebral infarction in patients with significant vascular diseases is termed multi-infarct dementia (MID; Hachinski et al. 1974). In previous studies, other terms used to describe MID included arteriosclerotic dementia, vascular dementia, and psychosis with cerebral arteriosclerosis. Unfortunately, diagnostic criteria have been hard to develop and have varied from study to study. However, longitudinal studies such as the Framingham study (Kase et al. 1989) employed more strict clinical criteria for the diagnosis of MID. These criteria included the use of the "Hachinski ischemic score" (Hachinski et al. 1975), brain imaging for confirmation of cerebral vascular disease, and documentation of onset of dementia only after one or more strokes. Ideally, a temporal relationship between stroke and dementia should be determined in order to diagnose MID.

MID can present a variety of different clinical syndromes. The most classic presentation is the patient who has multiple strokelike episodes, multifocal neurological signs, and CT or MRI evidence for multiple strokes. However, other patients (particularly those with chronic hypertension and diabetes) develop multiple subcortical strokes involving the basal ganglia, internal capsule, thalamus, and brain stem. Many of these patients will develop a slowly progressive subcortical symptom complex (Fisher 1982; Roman 1987; Wallin et al. 1991). In part because of the variability in the patterns of expression, MID can be mistaken for other dementing conditions. Conversely, in a substantial number of patients diagnosed with MID, AD changes are also present at postmortem examination (Thal et al. 1991).

Epidemiology of MID. MID is the second commonest cause for dementia in most countries (see Table 13–2). In the United States, it accounts for 12%–20% of dementia cases, although a more recent review suggested that 10% may be a more realistic estimate for prevalence (Kase 1991). Much higher rates have been shown in studies performed in Japan (48%–72%; Jorm et al. 1987; Shibayama et al. 1986), Finland (39%; Sulkava et al. 1985), and Italy (35%; Rocca et al. 1990). Some of these differences may relate to differences in the prevalence of hypertension, whereas others may have a strong genetic basis.

The true prevalence of MID or vascular dementia has been controversial. Some argue that this is an underdiagnosed entity (O'Brien 1988); others believe that it is overdiagnosed (Brust 1988). As with other dementia syndromes, the range of percentages may result from use of the different diagnostic criteria or age or gender distributions in various populations studied. Because advancing age and possibly lower levels of education are significant risk factors for AD and MID, overlapping clinical variables or coexisting diseases render accurate diagnosis impossible in some cases. Gender differences show a reverse trend in MID as compared to AD; a higher prevalence of MID is found in males as compared to females in all but one study (Jorm et al. 1987).

Studies conducted in Chinese communities showed wide variations in the rate of MID. It represented 27% of all dementia cases in Shanghai (Zhang et al. 1990), 54% in Beijing (Li et al. 1989), 64% in Singapore (Kua 1991), and 76% among residents with dementia in a Chinese-American nursing home in New York (Serby et al. 1987). These studies support a high prevalence of vascular dementia in Asian populations, although different methods for diagnosis probably best explain these wide variations. Additionally, some of these differences in prevalence may be explained by the different age distribution of the population; for example, the Beijing and Singapore populations were much younger than the Shanghai population. This emphasizes the need to perform age-adjusted analysis of prevalence in the epidemiological surveys.

Overall, studies performed with Chinese, Japanese, African-

American, and Italian subjects show a significantly higher proportion of MID patients compared to Caucasian Americans and Caucasian Europeans. In a study with postmortem confirmation of diagnosis of dementia in 144 of 6,000 autopsies performed at Johns Hopkins Hospital, there was a 23% prevalence of MID in African-Americans ($n = 15$) compared to 5% of MID in Caucasians ($n = 4$; de la Monte et al. 1989). Whether the percentages represent the differences in their genetic makeup or their cultural/dietary influences remains unknown.

Parkinson's Disease

The clinical syndrome. There are many different causes for parkinsonian syndromes, the commonest being idiopathic PD. A deficit of the dopaminergic system produces a complex of symptoms including tremor, rigidity, postural instability, decreased movement, and in some instances dementia. There are many causes for PD, including infection, intoxication, vascular disease, and degenerative diseases. However, most patients with PD have the degenerative idiopathic type. In patients with classic PD, a small subset (10%–15%) seem to have a familial form, but no genetic basis have been established (Ward et al. 1983). In addition, there are several disorders that have parkinsonism associated with other pathologies and are termed parkinsonism-plus syndromes. These include olivopontocerebellar degeneration, Shy-Drager syndrome, striatonigral degeneration, progressive supranuclear palsy, the ALS/PD complex of Guam, and the motor system degeneration syndrome found in the Azores. Clearly, parkinsonism can result from multiple etiologies. However, for the purpose of this discussion, we will focus on the dementia associated with PD and its epidemiology.

The prevalence of dementia associated with PD from a review of 17 studies is 35% (Brown and Marsden 1984). However, cognitive impairment has been reported to occur in as many as 85% of PD patients (McDowell and Cedarbaum 1986). The cognitive decline may occur early in the disease and is often insidious and progressive. In the past, some researchers have suggested that the dementia associated with PD is due to the co-occurrence of PD and AD. More recent work suggests that many patients with the co-occurrence of dementia and parkinsonism have a pathology that demonstrates Lewy bodies in the cortex (Lewy-body dementia). Biochemical changes in patients with PD and dementia show reduced levels of the enzyme choline acetyltransferase levels and decreased cell counts in the basal nucleus of Meynert, which suggests some overlap with the pathological changes of AD (Boller et al. 1980; Whitehouse et al. 1983). These overlapping abnormalities suggest similar pathogenic mechanisms may be involved in both of these common neurological diseases.

Epidemiology of PD. The prevalence of PD exceeds 100 per 100,000 in most studies performed in the United States, New Zealand, Australia, and northern Europe (see Table 13–3). However, some studies have shown that blacks have a lower incidence of PD than Caucasians (Kessler 1971, 1972; Reef 1977), whereas a more recent community survey performed in a biracial population in the United States (Copiah County, Mississippi) showed no substantial differences in prevalence regarding sex or race (Schoenberg et al. 1985a, 1985b). A further comparison of the black population in Copiah with the black population in Igbo-Ora, Nigeria—both rural regions—showed a surprising difference in age-adjusted prevalence: 341 versus 67 per 100,000, respectively (Schoenberg et al. 1988).

As with the studies in African countries, surveys in Asian countries such as Japan (Harada et al. 1983) and China (Li et al. 1985) also suggest a lower prevalence of PD. To account for these differences, one explanation included that postencephalitic parkinsonism was rare in Japan. In general, PD is more prevalent with more advanced age, among males more than females, and among Caucasians more than Asians or blacks. Whether these differences are due to either cultural-environmental variations and/or racial-genetic differences remains to be determined.

Although some of these studies have suggested the importance of genetic factors in the pathogenesis of PD, twin studies have shown low concordance rates in more than one region (Duvoisin et al. 1981; Marttila and Rinne 1976; Marttila et al. 1988; Ward et al. 1983). Coupled with the statistics in the different prevalence from African-Americans versus African blacks, as described previously, environmental causes appear more likely. In

1983, 1-methyl-4-phenyl-1,2,3,6-tetrahydropyridine (MPTP) was found to be a human neurotoxin producing a syndrome almost identical to PD (Ballard et al. 1985). Since that time, hypotheses for environmentally produced MPTP-like neurotoxin were

Table 13–3. Prevalence of Parkinson's disease in different countries

Country	Authors	Prevalence[a] (per 100,000)	Population and/or methods
Australia Victoria	Jenkins 1966	85	Physician referrals from Gippsland
China (People's Republic)	Li et al. 1985	44	Survey in six cities
England			
Carlisle	Brewis et al. 1966	113	Hospital and physician records
Leeds	Garland 1952	60	Postal survey of local practitioners
Finland	Marttila and Rinne 1976	120	Records from central statistics and local referrals
Iceland	Gudmundsson 1967	163	Review of all medically related sources
Italy (Sardinia)	Rosati et al. 1980	66	Mediterranean mixed European & African
Japan	Harada et al. 1983	81	Hospital records and insurance receipts
Nigeria	Osuntokun et al. 1987	59	Door-to-door survey of a town (pop. 20,000)
New Zealand Wellington	Pollock and Hornabrook 1966	106	Hospital, nursing homes, and local referrals
Sweden	Mjones 1949	160	Survey of special clinics
	Broman 1963	68	A 5-year hospital survey in Göteborg
United States			
Rochester, MN	Kurland 1958	157	Defined community records
Baltimore, MD	Kessler 1972	C = 125, B = 21	Community referral
Copiah, MS	Schoenberg et al. 1985b	C = 159, B = 103	Entire town (door-to-door) survey

Note. C = Caucasians; B = blacks.
[a] Observed Prevalence Ratio.

sought, but none have been found (Tanner 1989). Some investigators hypothesized that the drinking of well water in the rural regions may have accounted for the higher incidence seen in rural Canada (Rajput et al. 1984); a similar experience was also reported from a Chicago medical center (Tanner 1985). Many other environmental risk factors including viral causes were hypothesized and have been well summarized by Schoenberg (1987).

Prion Disease

Clinical characteristics. Prion disease is actually a group of diseases caused by an accumulation of an abnormal protein product for which Prusiner and colleagues (1987) coined the term "prion." There is a progressive spongiform degeneration of the nervous system typically leading to death within 1 year from the initial onset of symptoms. It is transmissible through inoculation of the infected tissue, which is resistant to routine sterilization techniques. The diseases affecting humans include *kuru* and CJD and a genetic form called Gerstmann-Straussler syndrome. In these conditions, definitive diagnosis can only be made with brain biopsy, which shows spongiform encephalopathy. Clinically, CJD patients initially present with vague symptoms such as fatigue and forgetfulness, but progress rapidly to dementia with aphasia and other cortical, pyramidal, extrapyramidal, and cerebellar signs, as well as myoclonus. In the final stages, these patients become stuporous, akinetic with decerebrate rigidity, myoclonus, and seizures.

Epidemiology of* kuru *and CJD. *Kuru* was the first prion disease described in comprehensive epidemiological studies (Gajdusek 1977). It occurred in the Fore tribe in Papua New Guinea and produced a spongiform encephalopathy. At the height of the prevalence, it affected 1% of the population and was the leading cause of death. The transmission was found to be due to the cannibalism of human brains during a mourning ritual. *Kuru* has largely disappeared with the cessation of cannibalism. CJD, however, is found to have a prevalence of 1 per million in the United States and abroad. A study in Israel showed a 30-fold greater prevalence in Jews of Libyan origin compared to Jews of European origin (Kahana et al. 1991). Initial studies erroneously speculated (as will be explained) that the incidence of CJD was due to the custom among Jews of North African and Middle Eastern origin of eating sheep eyeballs and brains, through which some contracted the disease through contamination by infected sheep tissue.

In the United States, transmissions of CJD have occurred in corneal transplants (Duffy et al. 1974) and growth hormone extracts from infected pituitary glands (Brown et al. 1985). Between 5% and 10% of CJD cases are familial, with an autosomal dominant inheritance pattern. Studies done in rural Czechoslovakia (Mitrova 1987) and among Libyan-born Jews living in Israel (Neugut et al. 1979; Zilber et al. 1991) showed high percentages (35%–47%) of familial cases, and 27% of the cases found in Chile were familial (Brown et al. 1987). These familial clusters have led to closer scrutiny of the genetic component of the disease.

As CJD became better understood through genetic studies of the prion protein, it was discovered that the high prevalence of CJD among Libyan Jews was due to a dominant point mutation in the prion protein gene (Hsiao et al. 1991). Similar point mutations occur in a familial variant of CJD called Gerstmann-Straussler-Scheinker (GSS) disease (Hsiao et al. 1991). These brilliant studies into these rare diseases exemplify how the use of careful epidemiological research, combined with powerful molecular genetic techniques, can lead to a clear understanding of the causes for a variety of dementia syndromes.

Western Pacific-ALS/PD-Dementia Complex

This syndrome characterized by ALS and a progressive parkinsonian-dementia syndrome was first recognized in 1947, when a high prevalence was described among peoples inhabiting scattered islands in the South Pacific (the Chamorros on the islands of Guam, Rota, and Tinian; Stanhope et al. 1972) and inhabitants on Kii Peninsula in Japan (Yase 1972). In these regions, prevalence rates were found of 50 per 100,000 for males and 20 per 100,000 for females; the male-to-female ratio was 1.8:1. More recently, a focus in New Guinea was discovered by Gajdusek (1979).

Initially, this syndrome was thought to be related to postencephalitic parkinsonism because of the clinical similarities between the two diseases (Mulder et al. 1954). After World War II, the incidence of the syndrome declined. This was attributed to improvements in general health and dietary care (Steele et al. 1990) on Guam. By 1972, the incidence had fallen by 50%. A more recent report (Garruto et al. 1986) suggested that calcium deficiency may have caused the deposition of toxic minerals in neurons, whereas the discovery of the neurotoxic cycad seed (Cycas circinalis) raised the possibility that a neurotoxin in this plant may have been the etiologic agent (Spencer et al. 1987). However, many researchers continue to explore the possibility of a viral cause for this syndrome (Gajdusek 1990; Hudson and Rice 1990). As with other dementia syndromes, careful epidemiologic studies will help to clarify and support the causative factors.

Frontal Lobe Degeneration

In recent years, there have been increasing interests in degenerative dementia affecting primarily the frontal lobe. This syndrome is also called "dementia of frontal lobe type" (Neary et al. 1988) and "frontal lobe dementia of non-Alzheimer type" (Gustafson et al. 1990; Miller et al. 1991). Patients afflicted with this syndrome typically present with social withdrawal or disinhibition and selective frontal and memory impairment, with relative sparing of attention, language, and visuospatial skills on neuropsychological testing. Cerebral blood flow studies also demonstrate frontal and temporal hypoperfusion, with relative sparing of parietal and occipital regions. Pathological studies showed Pick's bodies, gliosis, and neuronal loss in the same regions (Brun and Gustafson 1989). In many cases the disease appears to be inherited as an autosomally dominant gene.

Interestingly, this condition is being recognized more frequently and has been associated with diseases such as ALS (Brun and Gustafson 1989). A Japanese series (Morita et al. 1987) of 34 cases of amyotrophy associated with presenile dementia showed pathological changes consistent with FLD and suggested that this may be a new disease entity. It is more likely that, as the syndrome is better understood and recognized, it will be found to be a major cause of dementia.

AIDS Dementia Complex

Clinical characteristics. This entity is also called human immunodeficiency virus (HIV) encephalitis, or HIV encephalopathy, implicating a direct brain infection from the virus. Chronic progressive cognitive loss may occur along with motor and behavior changes, such as extremity weakness and apathy with personality changes. A subcortical dementia with psychomotor slowing characterizes these patients; they eventually become mute and bedridden. Many questions exist concerning the neuropathological, neuroimaging, and biochemical changes seen in these patients and the clinical syndrome.

Epidemiology of AIDS dementia complex. Before 1981, only 79 cases of AIDS were diagnosed in the United States and reported to the Centers for Disease Control (CDC). This number has reached an epidemic proportion of 226,281 cases in adults and 3,898 cases in children in the United States a decade later (CDC 1992). Statistics from the World Health Organization (WHO) and CDC indicate the United States has the highest number of reported cases, with Africa (including cases in 46 countries) second. These reported values reflect availability of HIV testing and medical assessment, systems of disease reporting, as well as actual differences in prevalence.

With the serologic diagnosis of AIDS, the incidence of this dementia has the potential of being more accurately assessed within the AIDS population. However, clouding of the statistics may arise from concurrent opportunistic infections affecting the central nervous system in these patients. A critique of 56 studies regarding approximately 800 subjects has shown that at some point following infection, an HIV-induced dementia is extremely common (Perry and Marotta 1987). More recently, a 10-year autopsy study in Switzerland of 345 AIDS patients showed 19% (n = 68) had morphological evidence of HIV encephalopathy (Kleihues et al. 1991), whereas another clinical study performed in Italy showed only 10% of 6,466 cases (n = 640) presented with

ADC (Chiesi et al. 1990). In the Italian study, the researchers attributed the decreased incidence to zidovudine (AZT) treatment, which had delayed the onset of ADC. Our understanding of this disease and the incidence of ADC is still evolving, and much research will be needed for better treatment strategies, as well as education for preventions.

FUTURE RESEARCH DIRECTIONS

The rich volume of data accumulated over the years provides a good basis for future research studies. Certain epidemiological factors, such as genetics and aging for AD and a rural predominance for PD, have emerged as important in various dementia syndromes. These clues help to focus research efforts into these conditions. The advent of powerful molecular genetic techniques may help to explain some of the differences in prevalence for the various dementing conditions. For example, better studies in genetics have helped to solve the puzzle of the Libyan-Jewish cluster of CJD cases, which was brought to attention by epidemiological studies. Continued studies in prevalence of MID and AIDS dementia will also help to focus preventive measures, such as education and perhaps a vaccine for HIV in the near future, in regions with higher prevalence.

As we discussed at the beginning of this chapter, there are still problems in diagnosis and study design in many dementia research projects. These will be key issues in future cross-cultural studies. Tightly controlled methodological procedures will be needed in the future; studies that compare prevalence in different regions need to use similar methods and to study comparable populations. As one of the greatest neuroepidemiologists, Bruce S. Schoenberg, put it: "The two most important considerations for the neuroepidemiologist are the representativeness of the population selected for investigation and the accuracy of the diagnoses in that population" (Schoenberg 1987, pp. 407–408).

REFERENCES

Ballard PA, Tetrud JW, Langston JW: Permanent human parkinsonism due to MPTP. Neurology 35:949–956, 1985

Boller F, Mizutani T, Roessmann V, et al: Parkinson disease, dementia and Alzheimer disease: clinico-pathological correlations. Ann Neurol 7:329, 1980
Boller F, Lopez OL, Moossy J: Diagnosis of dementia: clinicopathologic correlations. Neurology 38:76–79, 1989
Bollerup TR: Prevalence of mental illness among 70-year-olds domiciled in nine Copenhagen suburbs. Acta Psychiatr Scand 51:327–339, 1975
Brayne C, Calloway P: An epidemiological study of dementia in a rural population of elderly women. Br J Psychiatry 155:214–219, 1989
Brewis M, Poskanzer DC, Rolland C, et al: Neurological disease in an English city. Acta Neurol Scand (suppl 24) 42:1–89, 1966
Broman T: Parkinson's syndrome, prevalence and incidence in Göteborg. Acta Neurol Scand (suppl 4) 39:95–101, 1963
Brown P, Gajdusek DC, Gibbs CJ Jr, et al: Potential epidemic of Creutzfeldt-Jakob disease from human growth hormone therapy. N Engl J Med 313:728–731, 1985
Brown P, Cathala F, Raubertas RF, et al: The epidemiology of Creutzfeldt-Jakob disease: conclusion of a 15-year investigation in France and review of the world literature. Neurology 37:895–904, 1987
Brown RG, Marsden CD: How common is dementia in Parkinson's disease? Lancet 1:1262–1265, 1984
Brun AE, Gustafson L: Frontal lobe dysfunction: the patho-anatomical background of dementia. Bull Clin Neurosci 54:68–72, 1989
Brust JCM: Vascular dementia is overdiagnosed. Arch Neurol 45:798–801, 1988
Centers for Disease Control: Statistics from the Centers for Disease Control. AIDS 6:1229–1233, 1992
Chen XS, Zhang JZ, Jiang ZN, et al: A psychiatric epidemiological survey on elderly in Beijing City. Chung Hua Shen Ching Ching Shen Ko Tsa Chih 20:145–148, 1987
Chiesi A, Agresti MG, Dally LG, et al: Decrease in notifications of AIDS dementia complex in 1989–1990 in Italy: possible role of the early treatment with Zidovudine. Medicina 10:415–416, 1990
Cook RH, Ward BE, Austin JH: Studies in aging of the brain, IV: familial Alzheimer disease: relation to transmissible dementia aneuploidy, and microtubular defects. Neurology 29:1402–1412, 1979
Cook RH, Schneck SA, Clark DB: Twins with Alzheimer's Disease. Arch Neurol 38:300–301, 1981
Copeland JRM, Dewey ME, Wood N, et al: Range of mental illness among the elderly in the community: prevalence in Liverpool using the GMS-AGECAT package. Br J Psychiatry 150:815–823, 1987

Creasey H, Jorm A, Longley W, et al: Monozygotic twins discordant for Alzheimer's disease. Neurology 39:1474–1476, 1989

Cummings JL, Benson DF: Dementia: A Clinical Approach. Woburn, MA, Butterworth, 1983

de la Monte S, Hutchins GM, Moore W: Racial differences in the etiology of dementia and frequency of Alzheimer lesions in the brain. J Natl Med Assoc 81:644–652, 1989

Duffy P, Wolff J, Collins G, et al: Possible person-to-person transmission of Creutzfeldt-Jakob disease. N Engl J Med 299:692, 1974

Duvoison RC, Eldridge R, Williams A, et al: Twin study of Parkinson disease. Neurology 31:77–80, 1981

Ellis WG, McCulloch JR, Corley CL: Presenile dementia in Down's syndrome: ultrastructural identity with Alzheimer's disease. Neurology 24:101–106, 1974

Endo H, Yamamoto T, Kuzuya F: HLA system in senile dementia of Alzheimer type and multi-infarct dementia in Japan. Archives of Gerontology and Geriatrics 5:51–56, 1986

Evans DA, Funkenstein HH, Albert M, et al: Prevalence of Alzheimer's disease in a community population of older persons: higher than previously reported. JAMA 262:2551–2556, 1989

Fisher CM: Lacunar strokes and infarcts: a review. Neurology 32:871–876, 1982

Folstein MF, Folstein SE, McHugh PR: "Mini-mental state": a practical method for grading the cognitive state of patients for the clinician. J Psychiatr Res 12:185–198, 1975

Fratiglioni L, Gurt M, Forsell Y, et al: Prevalence of Alzheimer's disease and other dementias in an elderly urban population: relationship with age, sex, and education. Neurology 41:1886–1892, 1991

Gajdusek DC: Unconventional viruses and the origin and disappearance of Kuru. Science 197:943–960, 1977

Gajdusek DC: A focus of high incidence amyotrophic lateral sclerosis and Parkinsonism and dementia syndromes in a small population of Auyu and Jakai people of southern West New Guinea, in Amyotrophic Lateral Sclerosis. Edited by Tsubaki T, Toyokura Y. Baltimore, MD, University Park Press, 1979, pp 287–305

Gajdusek DC: Cycad toxicity not the cause of high-incidence amyotrophic lateral sclerosis/parkinsonism-dementia on Guam, Kii Peninsula of Japan, or in West New Guinea, in Amyotrophic Lateral Sclerosis: Concepts in Pathogenesis and Etiology. Edited by Hudson AJ. Toronto, Ontario, University of Toronto Press, 1990, pp 317–325

Garland HJ: Parkinsonism. BMJ 1:153–155, 1952

Garruto RM, Swyt C, Yanagihara R, et al: Intraneuronal co-localization of silicon with calcium and aluminum in amyotrophic lateral sclerosis and parkinsonism with dementia of Guam. New Engl J Med 315:711–712, 1986
Goudsmit JAAP, White BJ, Weitkamp LR, et al: Familial Alzheimer's disease in two kindreds of the same geographic and ethnic origin: a clinical and genetic study. J Neurol Sci 49:79–89, 1981
Gudmundsson KR: A clinical survey of parkinsonism in Iceland. Acta Neurol Scand (suppl 33) 43:9–60, 1967
Gustafson L, Brun A, Risberg J: Frontal lobe dementia of non-Alzheimer type, in Alzheimer's Disease (Advances in Neurology Series, Vol 51). Edited by Wurtman RJ, Corkin S, Growdeon J, et al. New York, Raven, 1990, pp 65–71
Hachinski VC, Lassen NA, Marshall J: Multi-infarct dementia: a cause of mental deterioration in the elderly. Lancet 2:201–210, 1974
Hachinski VC, Iliff LD, Zilhka E, et al: Cerebral blood flow in dementia. Arch Neurol 32:632–637, 1975
Harada I, Nishikawa S, Takahashi K: Epidemiology of Parkinson's disease in a Japanese city. Arch Neurol 40:151–154, 1983
Hay JJ, Ernst RL: The economic costs of Alzheimer's disease. Am J Public Health 77:1169–1175, 1987
Heston LL, Mastri AR, Anderson VE, et al: Dementia of the Alzheimer type: clinical genetics, natural history, and associated conditions. Arch Gen Psychiatry 38:1085–1090, 1981
Hsiao K, Meiner Z, Kahana E, et al: Mutation of the prion protein in Libyan Jews with Creutzfeldt-Jakob disease. N Engl J Med 324:1091–1097, 1991
Hudson AJ, Rice GPA: Similarities of Guamanian ALS/PD to Post-encephalitic Parkinsonism/ALS: possible viral cause. Can J Neurol Sci 17:427–433, 1990
Jenkins AC: Epidemiology of parkinsonism in Victoria. Med J Aust 2:496–502, 1966
Joachim CL, Morris JH, Selkoe DJ: Clinically diagnosed Alzheimer's disease: autopsy results in 150 cases. Ann Neurol 24:50–56, 1988
Jorm AF, Korten AE, Henderson AS: The prevalence of dementia: a quantitative integration of the literature. Br J Psychiatry 150:815–823, 1987
Kahana E, Ziller N, Abraham M: Do Creutzfeldt-Jakob disease patients of Jewish Libyan origin have unique clinical features? Neurology 41:1390–1392, 1991
Karasawa A, Kawashima K, Kasahara H: Epidemiological study of the senile in Tokyo metropolitan area, in World Psychiatric Association

Regional Symposium. Edited by Ohashi H, Nakayama K, Saito M, et al. Tokyo, Japan, The Japanese Society of Psychiatry and Neurology, 1982, pp 285–289

Kase CS: Epidemiology of multi-infarct dementia. Alzheimer Dis Assoc Disord 5:71–76, 1991

Kase CS, Wolf PA, Bachman DL, et al: Dementia and stroke: the Framingham study, in Cerebrovascular Disease, Sixteenth Research (Princeton) Conference. Edited by Ginsberg MD, Dietrich WD. New York, Raven, 1989, pp 193–197

Kay DWK, Beamish P, Roth M: Old age mental disorders in Newcastle upon Tyne, part I: a study of prevalence. Br J Psychiatry 110:146–158, 1964

Kessler I: Epidemiologic studies of Parkinson's disease, II: a hospital-based survey. Am J Epidemiol 95:308–318, 1971

Kessler I: Epidemiologic studies of Parkinson's disease, III: a community-based survey. Am J Epidemiol 96:242–254, 1972

Kleihues P, Leib SL, Strittmatter C, et al: HIV encephalopathy: incidence, definition and pathogenesis—results of a Swiss collaborative study. Acta Pathologica Japonica 41(3):197–205, 1991

Kohmen E, Beard CM, Offord KP, et al: Prevalence of medically diagnosed dementia in a defined United States population: Rochester, Minnesota, January 1, 1975. Neurology 39:773–776, 1989

Kua EH: The prevalence of dementia in elderly Chinese. Acta Psychiatr Scand 83:350–352, 1991

Kurland LT: Epidemiology: incidence, geographic distribution and genetic considerations, in Pathogenesis and Treatment of Parkinsonism. Edited by Fields WS. Springfield, IL, Charles C Thomas, 1958, pp 5–49

Leedom L, Miller BL: CT, MRI and NMR spectroscopy in the diagnosis of Alzheimer disease, in Diagnosis of Alzheimer's Disease. Edited by Giacobini E, Becker R. New York, PJ Taylor, 1990, pp 287–313

Li G, Schoenberg BS, Wang CC, et al: Prevalence survey of Parkinson's disease and other movement disorders in the People's Republic of China. Arch Neurol 42:655–657, 1985

Li G, Shen YC, Chen CH, et al: An epidemiological survey of age-related dementia in an urban area of Beijing. Acta Psychiatr Scand 79:557–563, 1989

Lin TY: A study of the incidence of mental disorder in Chinese and other cultures. Psychiatry 16:313–336, 1953

Liu CK, Miller BL, Cummings JL, et al: A quantitative MRI study of vascular dementia. Neurology 42:138–143, 1992

Marttila RJ, Rinne UK: Epidemiology of Parkinson's disease in Finland. Acta Neurol Scand 53:81–102, 1976

Marttila RJ, Kaprio J, Koskenvuo M, et al: Parkinson's disease in a nationwide twin cohort. Neurology 38:1217–1219, 1988
McDowell FH, Cedarbaum JM. Sixteen-year follow-up of 100 patients begun on levodopa in 1968: emerging problems. Adv Neurol 45:469–472, 1986
McKhann G, Drachman D, Folstein MF, et al: Clinical diagnosis of Alzheimer's disease: report of the NINCDS-ADRDA Work Group under the auspices of the Department of Health and Human Services Task Force on Alzheimer's disease. Neurology 34:939–944, 1984
Miller BL, Mena I, Daly J, et al: Temporal-parietal hypoperfusion with single-photon emission computerized tomography in conditions other than Alzheimer's disease. Dementia 1:41–45, 1990
Miller BL, Cummings JL, Villanueva-Meyer J, et al: Frontal lobe degeneration: clinical, neuropsychological and SPECT characteristics. Neurology 41:1374–1382, 1991
Mitrova E: Epidemiological analysis of Creutzfeldt-Jakob disease in Slovakia (1972–1985), in Virus Non Conventionnels du Système Nerveux Central. Edited by Court L. Paris, Masson, 1987
Mjones H: Paralysis agitans. Acta Psychiatrica et Neurologica Scandinavica Supplement 54:1–195, 1949
Molsa PK, Marttila RJ, Rinne UK: Epidemiology of dementia in a Finnish population. Acta Neurol Scand 65:541–552, 1982
Morita K, Kaiya H, Ikeda T, Namba M: Presenile dementia combined with amyotrophy: a review of 34 Japanese cases. Archives of Gerontology and Geriatrics 6:263–277, 1987
Mortimer JA: Alzheimer's disease and senile dementia: prevalence and incidence, in Alzheimer's Disease. Edited by Reisberg B. New York, Free Press, 1983, pp 144–148
Mulder DW, Kurland LT, Iriarte LLG: Neurologic diseases on the Island of Guam. U.S. Armed Forces Medical Journal 5:1724–1739, 1954
Neary D, Snowden JS, Northen B, Goulding P: Dementia of frontal lobe type. J Neurol Neurosurg Psychiatry 51:353–361, 1988
Nee LE, Polinsky RJ, Eldridge R, et al: A family with histologically confirmed Alzheimer's disease. Arch Neurol 40:2032–2038, 1980
Nee LE, Eldridge R, Sunderland T, et al: Dementia of the Alzheimer type: clinical and family study of 22 twin pairs. Neurology 37:359–363, 1987
Neugut RH, Neugut AI, Kahana E, et al: Creutzfeldt-Jakob disease: familial clustering among Libyan-born Israelis. Neurology 29:225–231, 1979
O'Brien MD: Vascular dementia is underdiagnosed. Arch Neurol 45:797–798, 1988

Osuntokun BO, Adeuja AOG, Schoenberg BS, et al: Neurological disorders in Nigerian Africans: a community-based study. Acta Neurol Scand 75:13–21, 1987

Payami H, Kaye J, Becker W, et al: HLA-A2, or a closely linked gene, confers susceptibility to early onset sporadic Alzheimer's disease in men. Neurology 41:1544–1548, 1991

Perry S, Marotta RF: AIDS dementia: a review of the literature. Alzheimer Dis Assoc Disord 1:221–235, 1987

Persson G: Prevalence of mental disorders in a 70-year-old urban population. Acta Psychiatr Scand 62:119–139, 1980

Pfeffer RI, Afifi AA, Chance JM: Prevalence of Alzheimer's disease in a retirement community. Am J Epidemiol 125:420–436, 1987

Pollock M, Hornabrook RW: The prevalence, natural history and dementia of Parkinson's disease. Brain 89:429–448, 1966

Prusiner SB, Gabizon R, McKinley MP: On the biology of prions. Acta Neuropathol (Berl) 72:299–314, 1987

Rajput AH, Stern W, Christ A, et al: Etiology of Parkinson's disease: environmental factors (abstract). Neurology 34(1):207, 1984

Rajput AA, Rozdilsky B, Rajput A: Accuracy of clinical diagnosis in parkinsonism—prospective study. Can J Neurol Sci 18:275–278, 1991

Reef HE: Prevalence of Parkinson's disease in a multiracial community, in Eleventh World Congress of Neurology. Edited by den Hartog Jager WA, Bruyn GW, Heijstee AJP. Amsterdam, Excerpta Medica, 1977, p 125

Rocca WA, Bonaiuto S, Lippi A, et al: Prevalence of clinically diagnosed Alzheimer's disease and other dementing disorders: a door-to-door survey in Appignano, Macerata Province, Italy. Neurology 40:626–631, 1990

Roman GC: Senile dementia of the Binswanger type: a vascular form of dementia in the elderly. JAMA 258:1782–1788, 1987

Rosati G, Granieri E, Pinna L, et al: The risk of Parkinson disease in Mediterranean people. Neurology 30:250–255, 1980

Salmon DP, Riekkinen PJ, Katzman R, et al: Cross-cultural studies of dementia: a comparison of mini-mental state examination performance in Finland and China. Arch Neurol 46:769–772, 1989

Schellenberg GD, Deeb SS, Boehnke M, et al: Association of an apolipoprotein CII allele with familial dementia of the Alzheimer type. J Neurogenet 4:97–108, 1987

Schoenberg BS: Environmental risk factors for Parkinson's disease: the epidemiologic evidence. Can J Neurol Sci 14:407–413, 1987

Schoenberg BS, Anderson DW, Haerer AF: Severe dementia: prevalence and clinical features in a biracial US population. Arch Neurol 42:740–743, 1985a

Schoenberg BS, Dallas WA, Haerer AF: Prevalence of Parkinson's disease in the biracial population of Copiah County, Mississippi. Neurology 35:841–845, 1985b
Schoenberg BS, Kokmen E, Okazaki H: Alzheimer's disease and other dementing illnesses in a defined United States population: incidence rates and clinical features. Ann Neurol 22:724–729, 1987
Schoenberg BS, Osuntokun BO, Adeuja AOG, et al: Comparison of the prevalence of Parkinson's disease in black populations in the rural United States and in rural Nigeria: door-to-door community studies. Neurology 38:645–646, 1988
Serby M, Chou JCY, Granssen EH: Dementia in an American-Chinese nursing home population. Am J Psychiatry 144:811–812, 1987
Shibayama H, Kasahara Y, Kobayashi H, et al: Prevalence of dementia in a Japanese elderly population. Acta Psychiatr Scand 74:144–151, 1986
Spencer PS, Nunn PB, Hugon J, et al: Guam amyotrophic lateral sclerosis-parkinsonism-dementia linked to a plant excitant neurotoxin. Science 237:517–522, 1987
St. George-Hyslop P, Tanzi TE, Polinsky RJ, et al: The genetic defect causing familial Alzheimer's disease maps on Chromosome 21. Science 235:885–890, 1987
St. George-Hyslop PH, Haines JL, Farer LA, et al: Genetic linkage studies suggest that Alzheimer's disease is not a single homogeneous disorder. Nature 347:194–197, 1990
Stanhope JM, Brody JA, Morris CE: Epidemiologic features of amyotrophic lateral sclerosis and Parkinsonism-dementia in Guam, Mariana Islands. Int J Epidemiol 1:199–210, 1972
Steele JC, Guzman TQ, Driver MG, et al: Nutritional factors in amyotrophic lateral sclerosis on Guam: observations from Umatac, in Amyotrophic Lateral Sclerosis: Concepts in Pathogenesis and Etiology. Edited by Hudson AJ. Toronto, Ontario, University of Toronto Press, 1990, pp 193–223
Sulkava R, Wikstrom J, Aromaa A, et al: Prevalence of severe dementia in Finland. Neurology 35:1025–1029, 1985
Tanner CM: Well water drinking and Parkinson's disease (abstract). Abstracts of the VIII International Symposium on Parkinson's Disease. New York, World Federation of Neurology Research Group on Extrapyramidal Diseases, 1985, p 11
Tanner CM: The role of environmental toxins in the etiology of Parkinson's disease. Trends Neurosci 12:49–54, 1989
Tanzi RE, St. George-Hyslop PH, Haines JL, et al: The genetic defect in familial Alzheimer's disease is not tightly linked to the amyloid B-protein gene. Nature 329:156–157, 1987

Terry RD, Katzman R: Senile dementia of the Alzheimer type. Ann Neurol 14:497–506, 1983

Thal L, Galasko D, Katzman R, et al: Patients assessed at an Alzheimer's center generally have Alzheimer pathology. Neurology 41:323, 1991

Treves T, Korczyn AD, Zilber N, et al: Presenile Dementia in Israel. Arch Neurol 43:26–29, 1986

Vinters H, Miller BL, Pardridge W: Brain amyloid and Alzheimer disease. Ann Intern Med 109:41–54, 1988

Wallin A, Blennow K, Gottfries CG: Subcortical symptoms predominate in vascular dementia. International Journal of Geriatric Psychiatry 6:137–145, 1991

Ward CD, Duvoisin RC, Ince SE, et al: Parkinson's disease in 65 pairs of twins and in a set of quadruplets. Neurology 33:815–825, 1983

Whitehouse PJ, Hedreen JC, White CL, et al: Basal forebrain neurons in the dementia of Parkinson's disease. Ann Neurol 13:243, 1983

Yase Y: The pathogenesis of amyotrophic lateral sclerosis. Lancet 2:292–296, 1972

Zhang M, Katzman R, Salmon D, et al: The prevalence of dementia and Alzheimer's disease in Shanghai, China: impact of age, gender, and education. Ann Neurol 27:428–437, 1990

Zilber N, Kahana E, Abraham M: The Libyan Creutzfeldt-Jakob disease focus in Israel: an epidemiologic evaluation. Neurology 41:1385–1389, 1991

Afterword

The preceding chapters comprehensively surveyed and summarized our current knowledge on how ethnic and cultural factors influence various aspects of psychopharmacology and psychobiology. As is evident from the wealth of information contained in this volume, progress in these relatively new research areas has been remarkable. The risk of oversimplification notwithstanding, we will attempt to provide a summary of some of this book's most important findings and conclusions.

1. Psychotropic responses, and more broadly, responses to pharmacological agents in general, are complex phenomena that are simultaneously influenced by biological, psychological, as well as sociocultural determinants. Interindividual variations in responses to most psychotropics (as well as nonpsychotropics) are substantial. Ethnicity represents one of the most important variables that contribute to such variations in drug response.
2. Various "nonbiological" factors, such as compliance and placebo response, are influenced by culturally determined beliefs and expectations. In addition, ethnic differences in pharmacokinetics and pharmacodynamics exist. Although some of these biologically based ethnic differences are genetically determined, others are caused by environmental factors such as diet and differential exposure to drug-inducing or drug-inhibiting agents in the environment.
3. Ethnic differences in pharmacokinetics have been observed between Asians and Caucasians with regard to haloperidol and some benzodiazepines, but not to lithium. The results involving tricyclic antidepressants (TCAs) have been inconsistent in this regard. In addition, pharmacodynamic factors and

Supported in part by Research Center on the Psychobiology of Ethnicity Grant MH47193 (Drs. Lin and Poland) and National Institute of Mental Health Research Scientist Development Award MH00534 (Dr. Poland).

plasma protein binding may also contribute to differences in psychotropic responses between these two ethnic groups. Fewer studies have focused on African-Americans and Hispanics. However, clinical and research data suggest that blacks in general may be more sensitive to TCAs and adinazolam for kinetic as well as dynamic reasons. Hispanics have been reported to require lower doses of TCAs for the clinical treatment of depression. In addition, significantly higher red blood cell (RBC)/plasma lithium ratio has been observed in blacks. However, the clinical significance of this phenomenon remains to be determined. Studies on cross-ethnic comparisons of tardive dyskinesia and other psychotropic side effects have thus far yielded inconsistent findings.

4. Aldehyde dehydrogenase deficiency and "flushing response" to alcohol among Asians, Alaska Natives, and American Indians represent the most dramatic and well-studied example of genetically determined ethnic differences in response to a psychoactive agent. Recent reports have also demonstrated a negative association between this trait and risk for the development of alcoholism.
5. Contrary to popular belief, ethnicity, culture, and psychobiology are not separate phenomena. On closer examination, their interactions are extensive and dynamic. In psychiatry, as well as other fields of medicine, ethnicity often is an important factor in disease susceptibility. There also are reasons to believe that environmental and cultural forces significantly influence neurodevelopment and possibly pathogenesis. These factors have major implications in our profession's search for "biological markers" for major psychiatric disorders, as well as for the "universality" of various psychiatric conditions.

Despite progress and achievement, many issues await clarification. To address these admittedly complicated issues, integrated research efforts with diverse designs and strategies will be needed. New techniques in pharmacogenetics should allow researchers to combine the genotyping and phenotyping of drug-metabolizing enzymes with traditional pharmacokinetic studies. The contribution of protein binding to ethnic and individual variations in drug responses could be further clarified by the simultaneous measurement of the free fractions of the drugs and their metabolites on the one hand, and the concentrations of plasma proteins involved in the binding of the drugs (such as the $alpha_1$ acid glycoproteins and albumins) on the other. In terms of pharmacodynamics, it is also very likely that advances in brain imaging technology will make it possible for researchers to directly assess drug-receptor interactions.

Similarly, progress in our understanding of the neurobiological correlates of psychiatric disorders will likely lead to the development of research tools that will not only benefit cross-ethnic/cross-cultural nosologic research, but will also contribute to the delineation of the "universal" aspects of various psychiatric syndromes. These exciting new advances in biotechnologies, combined with developments in clinical and cross-cultural psychiatric research methodologies, will ensure that the field will progress at an increasingly accelerated fashion. We hope that, by compiling this book, we have provided some impetus toward facilitating progress in this field.

Keh-Ming Lin, M.D., M.P.H.
Russell E. Poland, Ph.D.

Index

Page numbers in **boldface** refer to tables or figures.